M000290375

# CONFESSIONS
## of a Plastic Surgeon

*Shocking Stories About Enhancing*
*Butts, Boobs, and Beauty*

# THOMAS T. JENEBY, MD
### Board Certified Plastic Surgeon

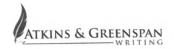
ATKINS & GREENSPAN
—— WRITING ——

For information about this title or to order other books
and/or electronic media, contact the publisher:

Atkins & Greenspan Writing
18530 Mack Avenue, Suite 166
Grosse Pointe Farms, MI 48236
www.atkinsgreenspan.com

ISBN
978-1-945875-70-0 (Hardcover)
978-1-945875-71-7 (Paperback)
978-1-945875-38-0 (eBook)

Printed in the United States of America

Cover and Interior design: Van-garde Imagery, Inc.

Front and Back Cover Photographs: ©Louis Scott Photography

All photographs used with permission.

NeoGraft, Cellfina, and CoolSculpting are registered trademarks.

# Dedication

*"Where there is charity and wisdom,*
*there is neither fear nor ignorance."*

—*Francis of Assisi*

I WOULD like to dedicate this book and a portion of all proceeds to the following charities which I hold dear to my heart.

To the following charities, I have given and will continue to give:

*Wounded Warrior Project, San Antonio*

*Family Violence Prevention Services (Formerly Battered Women and Children), San Antonio*

*Dress for Success San Antonio*

I believe that as Plastic Surgeons, we can contribute to the people and families within our community and make a difference with our *hands*, as well as with our wallets!

# Acknowledgments

*"I learned that courage was not the absence of fear
but the triumph over it.
The brave man is not he who does not feel afraid,
but he who conquers fear."*

—*Nelson Mandela*

I'd like to thank the following people for their enormous contribution to helping me stay sane throughout my life, both during periods of extreme joy and sometimes intense frustration. Being a Plastic Surgeon and becoming a Plastic Surgeon are a big deal and I never take it for granted. These people have helped keep me grounded.

My family: my mom, Dr. Lamya Alarif; my dad, Thamir AlHashimi; my sister, Michelle Resha Jeneby, Esq.; and my niece, Kenzie McConnell.

My friends, Dr. Wayne Lee; Dr. Herman Williams (for helping me find my wonderful writers) and getting me to write this book; Billy Madison; Derek Allgood; Nathan Williams; Felix Diaz; Mike Parsley; Dr. Eduardo Sanchez; Dr. Anand Thakur; Dr. Michael Pulizzi; Dr. Ricardo Alvarado; Dr. Mirhassan Farivar; Dr. Jorge Rincon; and Dr. Robert Green.

I have much gratitude for Elizabeth Ann Atkins and Catherine M. Greenspan of Atkins & Greenspan Writing for helping me bring this book to life.

I would also like to thank my entire staff at the Plastic and Cosmetic Center and Spa Black. These girls can be tireless angels as well as perfect examples of why tigers eat their young!

Ultimately, I would love to thank my wife, Ashliegh Thormann Jeneby, who is a one-in-a-billion, and my stepdaughter, Kallie.

# Foreword

We are living in a world obsessed with beauty and youth. Some would say too obsessed. The fashion and cosmetics industry thrive on this obsession. Treatments to enhance the appearance of the body and face, both surgical and non-surgical, are everywhere, and it seems they are multiplying by the hour.

Recently, as I walked out of the locker room of the club where I swim laps for fitness, I overheard a group of 12- to 14-year-old girls discussing the difference between liposuction and freezing fat. I cannot remember that ever happening when I was in junior high.

There is no question that plastic surgery has benefited from the obsession with appearance that seems to be so prominent in the modern world. In this book, Thomas Tayf Jeneby, MD takes the reader behind the scenes into the mind, heart, and soul of a busy plastic surgery practice. The reader comes to understand the pride, joy, and true pleasure that most of our patients give us when they entrust their bodies and faces to our skilled minds and well-trained hands to have surgical magic worked on them and transform them. He also speaks with honesty about the pain a few patients cause us when we fail to recognize their psychiatric issues before we operate on them and find that the surgical changes have not helped them, and in some cases, made them worse.

His discussions on marketing are cutting-edge. Not all Plastic Surgeons would agree with his approach but broadcasting live on the internet from your operating room certainly does educate patients about what plastic surgery is and is not. Watching liposuction live while it happens lets you know it is not a trip to the beauty parlor. Rather, plastic surgery is an invasion, an altering of anatomy with the goal of making a human being look normal in the case of reconstructive surgery, and better or different in the case of cosmetic surgery.

In all cases, setting expectations in the pre-operative consultation and communicating with the patient about what they can expect afterwards are just as important as performing well in the operating room. Dr. Jeneby brings these ideas to the fore in his unique way. Marketing is, after all, just letting the public know what you do and setting yourself apart from others who do the same thing in your unique way.

I have known Dr. Jeneby since his medical school days, when I met him while giving him his oral exam during his medical school clerkship. After reading this book, you will know him, too. Like me, you will find that he surprises you, entertains you, and most importantly informs you of what it is like for him to be a busy Plastic Surgeon today. His experience is not universal to all of us who have the pleasure to work in this field. It is uniquely Tayf's. I can promise you, after reading this book, you will never think of plastic surgery quite the same way again.

Isaac L. Wornom III, MD, FACS
Richmond Plastic Surgeons

# Preface

I am grateful to have had exceptional mentors at the University of Pennsylvania Division of Plastic Surgery: Dr. Isaac Wornom, Dr. Linton Whitaker, Dr. Scott Bartlett, the late Dr. Don LaRossa, Dr. David Low, Dr. Ben Chang, Dr. Lou Bucky, and Drs. Noone, Lohner, and Murphy.

This book is meant to entertain as well as provide information on what it's like in my office. It is written in a flowing and non-technical nature so as to appeal to all types of readers. I have changed some of the stories to remain HIPAA compliant, and any actual resemblances are purely coincidental.

The truth is: *These things happen to most of us in this field.*

# Contents

# Introduction

My shoes are covered with blood, chunks of fat, and scraps of skin.

I should have worn shoe "booties" when I dashed into the OR at 5:30 this morning.

But bloody shoes are the least of my worries as I insert my gloved hands into the hip-to-hip incision that I've cut in our patient's abdomen where I'm removing *29 pounds* of fat and skin.

This massive tummy tuck includes liposuction, and it's a big job. No worries, though, because my two surgical assistants, my nurse, and my anesthesiologist are rockin' it. Literally, to the beat of hip-hop/R&B music that's pulsing over the sterile blue surgical draping that covers everything except our patient's gaping incision.

I'm literally elbow-deep in this five-hour, blood-and-fat fest, and my stomach is growling. But at the moment, I can neither eat nor answer nature's call to go to the bathroom.

Because I'm a board-certified Plastic Surgeon specializing in plastic and cosmetic surgery and doing what I love requires total focus. I've been mastering the art of sculpting bodies to make them more beautiful in the eyes of their beholders for more than 18 years. This art gives me the power to transform lives. And I have a blast doing it.

But my life is beyond crazy.

As soon as I complete a hopefully "flawless" (easier said than done) procedure and seamlessly stitch up this patient—who will wake up with a dramatically improved appearance and life—I step out of the sanctuary of my private OR, and I'm confronted by the sheer *insanity* of my daily reality.

"Dr. Jeneby, this nipple is two millimeters lower than the other nipple!" a furious patient yells as I enter her room for a consultation. It's been several weeks since her surgery for a breast augmentation, or breast aug for short.

"You're healing perfectly," I assure her, "and your breast aug is beautiful. There's no obvious difference in your nipples."

"One is lower!" she shouts. "They're uneven. I can see it when I'm naked. You have to fix this!"

I always try to keep my cool, and patient satisfaction is paramount. So, I say, "Alright, let's schedule you to come back in. In nine to 12 months, if this is still apparent, I will take care of that."

*WTH,* I think, *even my nipples are uneven.*

Time is ticking, and I have multiple patients to see before the next surgery. I hurry into the black, marbled hallway that's lined with framed awards and magazine covers featuring me and my Joint Commission Credentialed Surgery Center and Spa: Spa Black.

As I rush toward the stairwell to meet another patient upstairs in Spa Black, I'm intercepted by one of my 21 female staff members, who can be nuts at any given moment.

*Oh, geez, what now?* I think.

"Dr. Jeneby," nurse Donna whispers in a conspiratorial tone. "Sheila was late today, and I think she's stealing Botox and doing Botox parties in her apartment with her friends who pay her for it!"

This reminds me of mafia movies: *Who's telling the truth? How do I find this out? Does Donna just not like Sheila, or is she stealing it herself? Geez!*

"Show me proof," I say. The last time this nurse tattled on someone, I saw her eating cookies with the alleged guilty party 10 minutes later. They hate each other one minute but are friendly to each other's faces the next. They laugh and even eat lunch together. How do they not like each other one minute and act like BFF's the next??? It's a maddening and never-ending saga of "Who's-gonna-tell-on-who so I look good for Dr. J?"

My staff has shown me all kinds of crazy, like when an angry boyfriend kidnapped my employee and locked her in the *trunk* of his car during business hours on my much-coveted, five-minute lunch break, nonetheless—and my staff tried to help the local police solve the crime.

On this day, I pray for peace and productivity as I zip up the steps to Spa Black, where we provide beauty treatments such as Botox, vaginal tightening, cellulite repair, CoolSculpting fat removal, fillers for lips and faces, facials, and microderms, to name a few.

"Dr. Jeneby!" my patient snaps when I enter the room.

The impressive "before" and "after" photos of her butt and thighs are illuminated on a lighted display board.

My technician stands beside the photos. She says, "You can see there's really dramatic improvement, thanks to the cellulite removal treatment we performed on her. But she's still not happy—"

"There are still some dimples!" shouts this 40-something patient who should be thrilled to now have a rear end that younger women would envy. "It's not smooth enough! You need to do more!"

I glance away from her furious face and study the "before" and "after" pics.

"To be perfectly honest," I say, "based on my 18 years of experience, you look amazing. This is pretty much as good as it gets. You're not going to look any better with more treatment."

Meanwhile, I'm thinking, *I am not an ironing board!*

She's shaking her head. "I'll sue you! Or give me a refund! If you don't, I'll tell every person I know not to come here!"

Threats are part of being in this field. After 18 years, I remain cool.

I am unfazed as I leave the room. Before the procedure, she signed a thick stack of consent forms. We provided exquisite service, with an excellent result, but she—and many of our patients—think I am a magician who can transform flaws into absolute perfection.

It's funny sometimes, when I'm interviewing a patient during a consult, I often say, "This is not going to be perfect; I'm a physician, not a magician."

The patient laughs, and says, "Oh, I don't expect perfection."

*Hmmm... Yes, you do!*

The bottom line is, this woman is part of the 20 percent of a Plastic Surgeon's patients who can make life a living hell because they are never happy. Some have Body Dysmorphic Disorder; others simply have unrealistic expectations. I'm used to it, so my mind whizzes forward.

"Let's try and make her as happy as humanly possible," I tell my staff.

Without missing a beat, another staff member calls out, "Dr. Jeneby, you're needed back downstairs!"

I zoom back downstairs to the clinic, where I perform a breast augmentation for a young woman. She's an exotic dancer, and she wants a dramatic enhancement. After surgery, a lot of these ladies have said they made their money back in *tips,* thanks to the implants, in two weeks! TWO WEEKS!! So, that's what we give her.

After the procedure, while she's in recovery, I'm going from room to room, meeting with patients.

They include a woman whose face was literally smashed during a domestic violence incident. I am going to reconstruct her face and restore her beauty and dignity at no charge. A camera crew films the consultation to showcase my special brand of philanthropy that involves donating my services to help domestic violence survivors.

Meanwhile, my staff consults with potential new clients. Men, women, and couples pack our lobby every day after hearing about boob jobs, butt lifts, lipo, tummy tucks, Mommy Makeovers, Daddy Makeovers, chest and ab sculpting, and much more after: hearing word-of-mouth recommendations; seeing my billboards around town; learning about us during live operations on Snapchat, Facebook, Instagram, and Twitter; following us on social media; watching me on national TV programs such as *Inside Edition*; and hearing me frequently on the nationally syndicated *Billy Madison Show*, one of San Antonio's top morning radio programs.

Suddenly, over the buzz of my staff talking with new patients and escorting them to consultation rooms, I hear the exotic dancer, who's supposed to be in recovery, shouting at the top of her lungs: "Look at my fucking tits!"

Her ecstatic voice echoes through the entire clinic, stopping everyone in their tracks. I hurry into the hallway.

People in the lobby are laughing and commenting about the happy patient, clearly a satisfied customer!

And I couldn't be more thrilled! What better advertising is there? *Welcome to my crazy world!*

I'm Thomas Jeneby, MD, a board-certified, Ivy League-educated Plastic Surgeon specializing in cosmetic surgery who founded the Plastic and Cosmetic Center of South Texas, Spa Black, and Palm Tree Surgi-Center.

If you had told me back when I was growing up as the son of immigrants in the Washington, DC area that this would be my life, I never would have believed you. But it was hard work to get here. After four years of college, I attended the Medical College of Virginia (Virginia Commonwealth University), where I was featured in the *top 10 percent of my class* and was president of the Medical Honor Society (AOA), an elite group of doctors worldwide. I did my residency in Combined General & Plastic Surgery at the Hospital of the University of Pennsylvania, where 300 Ivy League applicants competed for two positions per year. I have extensive training in both adult and pediatric plastic surgery, and I earned a 91 percent score on my recertification in 2012 with the American Board of Plastic Surgery.

I love what I do!

No question about it, I'm eccentric. I have long hair, speak my mind, and wear attention-grabbing clothes and cowboy boots. I love being the long-haired guy in the room! And, the hair even books surgeries!

I wrote this book to give you an exclusive peek into the fascinating world of plastic surgery through the eyes of an eccentric doc who tells it like it is. Yes, there are curse words and funny tales in this book. What I do is fascinating and sexy. But behind the scenes, it can be maddening.

In this book, you'll read stories that will show you what it's like to go through all the schooling and have a wonderful, booming practice, while those 20 percent of patients wreak havoc on my mind.

Sometimes it's so bad: *Oh, what the hell was I thinking, becoming a Plastic Surgeon? I want to throw up on myself and swallow my own vomit.*

My friends and colleagues joke all the time at national meetings about how social media has made things both better *and* worse.

My goal is to give you a peek into the daily reality of being a Plastic Surgeon specializing in cosmetic surgery. So, get ready to hear some shocking secrets about enhancing butts, boobs, and beauty.

Thomas T. Jeneby, MD
Board Certified Plastic & Cosmetic Surgeon
The Plastic and Cosmetic Center of South Texas
Palm Tree Surgi-Center and Spa Black

# 1

# Just Call Me a Psychiatrist
# with a Scalpel

*"Crazy people don't sit around
wondering if they're nuts."*

—*Jake Gyllenhaal*

Hey, you're looking beautiful!" I playfully call to my recovering patient in the PACU (Post Anesthesia Care Unit) in my private OR. "The Playboy Mansion called. They're sending the jet!" I get a lot of smiles for that.

Hip-hop music booms, and my every move is airing live on Facebook and Snapchat. Viewers everywhere have just watched me perform a breast augmentation using my specialty: *adjustable breast implants*. Today I enhanced a young lady from her natural size of a B-cup to a more voluptuous C-cup.

"Thirty-nine minutes!" announces my lead surgical tech, Jetsy, who is like my right hand in the OR. We've done so many of these procedures, and I've thrown nearly half a million sutures in 18 years, so it's second nature to seamlessly stitch up the incisions beneath this patient's breasts.

The beauty of adjustable saline breast implants is that she can now go bigger and bigger over time, which is far less traumatic than the traditional process of having large implants inserted as a one-shot deal that shocks the body with enormous swelling, horrible pain and soreness, and creates very large stretch marks.

The way adjustable implants work is this: I insert empty silicone sacs attached to a port, then pump in saline fluid to increase her breast size. Now, the port (which is under the skin and not visible) can be accessed for the next several months, so we can gradually pump in more saline and increase the size. I eventually remove the port through the same incision under local anesthesia in 5 to 10 minutes. People who get them are so impressed, they send their friends, who also love them.

This woman was a great patient from the start. She knew what she wanted, and she was getting a breast aug for herself. She asked the right questions, and followed our instructions to a T. We love that, because believe me, that is not the norm.

"Perfect, just perfect," I say as I dash toward the door. It's only 9:00 a.m., and I don't want to leave the sanctuary of my operating room. It's so peaceful, and I'm doing what I love most. But in order to keep the patients coming in for plastic and cosmetic surgeries, I have to do consults with new people and manage my 21 employees who keep the Plastic and Cosmetic Center of South Texas and Spa Black running like clockwork.

"Thanks, Dr. Flores!" I call to my anesthesiologist, who's been monitoring the patient's general anesthesia and vitals during the procedure. We get along great—she's like a second sister to me and is very opinionated! She is super bright and loves to talk about anything and everything.

She raises her head and nods from behind the curtain that blocks the patient's face from me and my nurses, as well as the cameras that broadcast live on social media (with the patient's permission, of course).

"Great job, everybody!"

I hurry out of the OR, remove my mask, latex gloves, and blue, sterile gown, then dash down the hall for consults.

These consultations are where I and my staff screen potential new patients to see if they're ready, willing, and able to undergo the procedures that they've come to talk about with us.

Unlike what some people may think, no one just walks in, pays the fee, and gets a procedure.

My decision to cut or not to cut depends on your lifestyle as well as your mental health and whether I believe you can take care of yourself after surgery the way I want you to! Over the years, I've become more selective as patients have become more demanding and their attention spans have shrunk!

Several other factors that you might think are unrelated to your desire to boost your beauty with bigger boobs, a Brazilian Butt Lift, a tummy tuck, liposuction, a Mommy Makeover, or any of the procedures that we offer at the Plastic and Cosmetic Center of South Texas, also come into play.

The mental health component of plastic surgery is HUGE! I sometimes consider myself a "psychiatrist who operates occasionally." I have to look into your *mind* before I can do anything with your *body*.

My staff works on the front lines of screening potential new patients to determine whether they are mentally, emotionally, and physically fit enough to endure our procedures and cope with the dramatic changes they will experience as a result.

*"Dr. J., this lady is cray-cray," my staff might say.*

*"She really is!"*

*"Please don't say yes! She will eat us alive!"*

The 21 women working in my plastic surgery center and spa in the two-story building that I own in San Antonio are experienced and have hawk-like instincts to spot off-the-wall traits.

Before I meet with potential patients, my staff provides a complimentary pre-consultation to assess them, look at their medical history, review their desired procedure, and provide a quote. If necessary, we need a psych evaluation if they're on anti-depressants and a cardiology evaluation if they're hypertensive. If they're on multiple meds, we tell them we need clearance from whomever is prescribing those meds.

I see the patient once they have been screened, *or else I'd go nuts.*

"Sometimes we get real crazy people, so we refer them to other doctors who can help them," says my clinical manager, Sylvia Montes.

Another way that we weed out unqualified individuals is by the sheer price of the procedure they're seeking. That usually scares them away.

But if they make it past my staff's initial screening, it's time for me to meet with them for an official consultation. I've got 10 to 20 minutes to assess whether they're a good candidate for plastic or cosmetic surgery. I might do these 30 times a day with new patients, so I have to be fast—and accurate.

During these consults, my mind is whizzing, and I am in the

zone. I need to do split-second evaluations from the moment I scoot into the exam room with one of my staff members.

"Hi, I'm Dr. Jeneby, thanks for coming!" I say, extending my hand to the 30-ish woman and a 40-ish man. She's wearing a form-fitting sundress, and he's in jeans and a polo shirt. Her handshake is weak and shaky, and she casts a timid look up at me with a tiny smile. His handshake is strong, and he sits back in the chair with a posture like he owns the place.

*He doesn't.*

*I do.*

During the first minute, I'm trying to figure out which of the four subsets of patients these folks fit into.

"So, you're here to talk about a breast augmentation," I say, looking directly into the woman's eyes. People who don't look back into your eyes are a potential red flag!

She glances at her husband first, who says, "Yeah, she's about a B-cup right now and *we* want to take her to double Ds."

*What's this "we" bullshhhhh...?*

As he talks, his phone beeps and he pulls it out of his pocket, glances at it. I can tell from his facial muscles that's he trying to suppress a sneaky smile like *he's probably getting a hot text from another woman* (which happens).

He glances at me, then back to his phone like he's sending a text.

I turn to the woman. "Tell me, in your own words, what do *you* want?"

"Um," she says, biting her bottom lip. Her eyes dart toward the man, who's completely ignoring us now. She looks back at me, and says, "Um, I want—um..."

I've been in the room less than a minute, and I can *guess* exactly what's going on here. I predict the following: She knows her husband is cheating, and she thinks that by getting bigger boobs, she can keep his attention. He seems like a real controlling jerk and is probably telling her that in order to make him stay with her, she'd better boost the boob size or else. This is one of the classic profiles of a potential patient, and I'll explain more later.

Meanwhile, I'm not getting a good feeling about this couple. Instead of the Plastic Surgeon's office, they should be heading to couples' counseling or divorce court.

She glances back at her husband, who is utterly engrossed with his phone.

"Don't look at him," I say to the woman. "Look at me and tell me what brings you here today. You're the one who will have to go under anesthesia, endure the pain, and take the risks! Plus, you'll need recovery time off work, and you'll need someone to take care of your two kids."

She nods and blinks. I stare at her and glance at him without blinking.

"Dude," I say to the man, who doesn't look up. "She won't be able to give them baths, change diapers, or lift them up for a while. You'll need to treat her like a princess and really help out around the house."

He shakes his head without looking up from the phone. "She can get her aunt to help with all that shit."

*I'm pissed.*

Sixty to seventy percent of infections and complications occur if you don't take care of yourself *post-operatively*.

I can literally see her shrink, and I can feel her angst. I don't care how much this guy wants to pay me, I don't perform surgeries in situations where I feel someone is being coerced or altering her body for the wrong reasons.

*Why are you really here?*

Then I notice her hand is shaking. I glance at her chart. "It says you're on anti-anxiety meds. How long have you been on those?"

She glances down shamefully.

The man huffs. "Why the hell did you put that on there? I told you they'd make a stink—"

*WOAH!* In my mind, this consult is over, and I'm saying, *Next!*

"We need to get a psych clearance from your doctor who prescribes those meds," I say. "Otherwise it's too risky to undergo a procedure."

I know this won't happen, and they won't be back.

Eight minutes have passed. I hurry into the next consult. This time it's a young woman, very pretty, wearing tight clothes and a lot of makeup. She's a little doughy through the middle, and her breasts look deflated.

"It's booby time!" she shrieks, excited to see me. "Dr. Jeneby, I just love you. I have three friends who came to you and they are so happy. I want you to fix my body now. I need a mega Mommy Makeover—lipo, tummy tuck, big boobs, and the BBL."

"Brazilian Butt Lift," I say. "You know that's where we take the fat we suction out of your abdomen and back through lipo, and insert it into your behind, so we create a whole new curvy contour for your entire body."

She shrieks. "Yes! Wheel me in now!"

"You're going for the whole shebang," I say, glancing at my assistant, who nods. That means this woman has the cash to pay for this expensive makeover.

She's looking me in the eyes. She's very clear on what she wants. And she seems to be doing this on her own. Intelligent, confident, and—

"Now let me explain what I'm going to do, and I need you to repeat it back to me," I say.

As I give the turbo-speed rundown of the procedures, she listens intently. "Now you—"

She spits it back at me, nearly word for word, and gives me a big smile.

*Bingo!*

"Let's get you on the schedule!"

"Wait, Dr. Jeneby," she says, "I read on Google that there's a risk of—"

*Shoot me now!* "There is no Dr. Google!" I exclaim playfully. "Do not go to Dr. Google! If you read the patient forums of people complaining about their Plastic Surgeon, 9.8 times out of 10, they had a hand in it. I've seen it. If you have any questions or problems, ask me directly. Okay?"

"Yes," she says. "I'll see you on operating day!"


## Psychology Rules

Fortunately, my staff includes someone with a master's degree in psychology who can spot offbeat patients before they even get a consult with me.

"Sometimes I tell Dr. Jeneby that I sense instability in the consults," says Anissa Snyder, one of my patient relation coordinators. "Maybe the men or women can't follow a conversation, won't make eye contact, can't sit still, or they talk in third person when referring to themselves. It's a red flag when someone says, 'What she would like is…' and I say, 'You mean, what you would like is…' to clarify. That could be waving a red flag for schizophrenia or a serious mental health disorder."

Anissa is the perfect person leading this crucial task, thanks to her bachelor's degree in psychology and a master's degree in psychological science, as well as years of teaching psychology at the University of Texas at San Antonio. Even better, she knows firsthand how we operate, because we first met when she came to me in 2013 for a breast augmentation and skin removal after she lost an incredible 234 pounds thanks to bariatric surgery.

Anissa and my other staff members who screen new patients use an extensive questionnaire to learn whether the potential new patients have any history of drug abuse, including pain killers that might have resulted from past surgeries or accidents.

Nancy is my "Latina coordinator" who primarily deals with the Hispanic population. She is one of the few in the office who speaks fluent *SURGICAL* Spanish (terms and points having to do with surgery). Living in South Texas—this is a REQUIREMENT! These patients are difficult if I don't get their inflections or their exact desires because of language barriers. Nancy helps me speak my Spanish like a pro!

Katrina is the youngest and quietest on staff but is resolute and is mainly my "millennial" coordinator. She is 25 and speaks millennial. *Yes, a millennial translator!*

I trust the judgment of all my patient relation coordinators.

"If they're recovering alcoholics or drug addicts and have addictive behaviors," Anissa says, "there's a risk that they might get addicted to plastic surgery because of Body Dysmorphic Disorder, which gives people a distorted perception of what they really look like. We've had patients affected by that. Dr. Jeneby did liposuction on the inside of a woman's knees and she looked great, but she was very unhappy with the results. People with BDD will have surgery after surgery and never be pleased with the results because they have an underlying psychological condition."

That is one fast track to hell that I and my staff want to avoid at all costs. Hence, the initial scrutiny.

Other indicators that someone is off?

"They can't sit still," Anissa says, "Or they're picking at their fingers or their scalp, they're very unsure of themselves, they talk with a hand over their mouth, which is a sign of deception, or they tell me a different story than what they tell Dr. Jeneby, or they don't seem like they can follow directions well."

Plastic and cosmetic surgery procedures involve following meticulous instructions before and after, and the patient's life can literally depend upon following these instructions. Oftentimes (60-70 percent), patients will reveal that they did not follow instructions as we discussed, or even better, their significant other "rats" on them.

For example, they are instructed not to take any medications that can have a blood-thinning effect prior to surgery. We're forced to cancel 10 percent of procedures because patients forget or aren't following simple pre-op instructions, even though we've provided these instructions in writing and reiterated them verbally multiple times. They take their birth control pills or a pain-relief medication or cocaine, amphetamine, marijuana, PCP, ecstasy... and BAM! It's in their system and could cause excessive and life-threatening bleeding or arrhythmias (heart issues) during surgery. So, we have to reschedule.

The patient also needs the mental and physical toughness for the potential of enduring pain, risking infection, and adjusting to a new look and feeling in their body. Can they handle changes in how people might respond to their new appearance? New boobs can turn heads and trigger a lot of attention; is this person ready for that?

In a nutshell, we evaluate potential patients in the following four categories on our questionnaire.

**Mental Health.** We ask if the patient is taking any antidepressants or mood-stabilizing medications. If so, we need to know for how long, who prescribed them, and we need that doctor to provide "clearance" for surgery. We also ask if the individual has had any major traumas within the past three months, such as divorce or death of a loved one. We do not operate if someone has a fresh emotional wound because these big turbulences have a tendency to skew judgments. Once a procedure is done, it's done.

**Physical Health.** This requires a full medical history that includes finding out whether an individual has health ailments that could make it risky to give them anesthesia during surgery. Do they, for example, have diabetes or high blood pressure or a heart condition that could cause a precarious situation under anesthesia?

**Listening Skills.** I quickly recite what the procedure will involve. Then I ask the potential patient to repeat what I said. Most cannot. *Frightening!*

**Lifestyle.** People who smoke or are morbidly obese or hint that they use illicit drugs and exhibit many other factors, can raise red flags that alert us that this person may not be a good candidate for physically enduring the rigors of plastic surgery.

Don't think we're being overly cautious or paranoid about this.

A ton of studies link major mental health problems to plastic surgery, and they raise the question of whether the chicken or the egg came first. Is someone who's mentally unstable more likely to want to dramatically change their body with surgery? Or is someone who has their body surgically altered prone to developing psychological problems? Either way, I want to avoid operating on people who could come back and bite me in the ass.

According to an article entitled "Mental Health Issues Worsen Following Cosmetic Surgery," published in *The Alternative Daily* on October 15, 2013: "Researchers found strong evidence that women with mental health issues were more likely to choose surgery; more had a history of psychological problems including depression and anxiety, increased instance of illicit drug use, suicide attempts, and self-harm. The surgery was found to do little to quell these issues, in fact in most cases they worsened." [1]

The co-author of the study noted that symptoms of depression, anxiety, excessive alcohol consumption, and eating disorders actually *increased.* [2]

The authors also found that: "...when life fails to improve following the change, mental health problems might worsen because of the disappointment." [3]

I don't need a study to tell me this; I already know it from 18 years of experience.

Obviously, plastic surgery is a life-altering phenomenon that can vastly improve a person's self-esteem, boost their vitality, attract a new husband or wife, and make magic happen in countless ways.

---

[1]  https://www.thealternativedaily.com/mental-health-issues-worsen-following-cosmetic-surgery/
[2]  https://www.thealternativedaily.com/mental-health-issues-worsen-following-cosmetic-surgery/
[3]  https://www.thealternativedaily.com/mental-health-issues-worsen-following-cosmetic-surgery/

## Beware of "Break-Away Boobs"

It sounds like a joke, but Break-Away Boobs are very real! They can *accelerate* romantic relationships and marriages or divorces into a danger zone with no point of return. Babies, too! I think of them like modern day rocket engines pushing their wearers into…dun dun dun….the unknown!

I've seen so many women get a breast augmentation, then immediately leave their husband or boyfriend in the dust. The woman's confidence spikes, she looks amazing, and she attracts a hot new boyfriend or girlfriend. Sometimes the biggest loser is the poor guy who may have paid six grand for the procedure.

Sometimes, however, it's me who has to make a fast break-away from a psychiatric nightmare who wants to be my patient. Just because someone can afford to pay—since our procedures are not covered by insurance—doesn't mean we're willing to do it. In fact, we refuse to provide procedures for about 20 to 30 percent of the men and women who come to our Center for free consultations.

"I can't help you," I tell them.

"What?" they ask. "You're the best!"

"I don't think I'm capable of making you happy," I say.

I've experienced certain personality types enough to recognize them right away.

When I meet them, it's like my gut flips on a giant red neon *NO!* sign that flashes in my head. In the worst cases, it's a straight-up, *AWWW, HELL NO!*

These people are not physically fixable because they are afflicted by a skewed perception of themselves and the people they blame for their problems. These are the types who, despite a perfect procedure, are impossible to please. And guess who gets blamed?

The doc!

"I don't like them," they might say about the beautiful breasts that I created for them.

"Your breasts are well within the standard of measurement and beauty norms," I tell them. "Would you please go and get a second opinion?"

"No," they answer. "I don't like what you did. They're uneven."

These types end up calling me a terrible surgeon—and worse. They threaten to sue, they write bad reviews online (from which I have zero recourse!), and they generally become what we call in the business a nightmare. Like the woman who ripped off her blouse, ran into our waiting room full of new patients, and screamed, "Look what this butcher did to me!" for a very minor difference in her breasts.

When I and my staff spot these personality types, we refuse to provide services.

On the other hand, some girls come in and are like, "Yeah, I can't wait! This is awesome!"

We get a lot of exotic dancers, and I have to gauge them as well.

The best patients know exactly what they want and what they're getting into, and they're willing to follow my instructions meticulously for a successful surgery and recovery.

My business is a numbers game. We bring in 1,200 people per year for consults and 500 make the cut to have surgery, which includes people who can get financing or whom we finance. To do this, every Tuesday, I see 15 to 20 new people who want to transform their bodies. My coordinators "interview" another 100 or so a week.

If the man or woman passes my staff's screenings, then they're scheduled for an appointment with me. Here's when the fun begins! Imagine, I'm in my black scrubs, dashing out of procedures, heading into patient rooms for consults. The day moves at lightning speed, as I try to meet with as many potential new patients as possible, and do a scrupulous job assessing them in roughly 15 to 20 minutes.

That's how long I have to decide if they're cuckoo. I'm making judgements in nanoseconds based on how they look, how they're talking, acting, listening (or not listening).

I've concluded that we see five types of women who get plastic surgery. (Men are a whole different ball game, and I'll talk about that later. Stay tuned.)

## Dr. Jeneby's Five Types of Women Who Get Plastic Surgery

**1. Very Happy.** She is the ideal patient. She's extremely happy, confident, and determined to go under the knife because she wants the facelift, the breast aug, the Brazilian Butt Lift, the tummy tuck, the Mommy Makeover. She's eager to follow instructions for the best possible surgery and outcome. She's expecting excellence from me but does not have unrealistic expectations about what surgery can and cannot do for her body. Her motive is simply to feel better about herself, for herself.

**2. About to Cheat.** This woman is unhappy with her significant other, and she's about to get her groove on with another man (or woman!). But first, she wants new boobs, a better booty, a tummy tuck, lipo, or maybe all of the above, all at once! Maybe her significant other hasn't been treating her right, or he's not giving her the attention she needs. But she's about to dramatically alter her body because she's got a plan to cheat on this dude and possibly break away with someone who will appreciate her.

**3. Cheating.** This woman is unhappy with her significant other and is currently cheating on him. Somehow, he pushed her into the arms of another man, and chances are, once she gets her procedure, Guy #1 is toast.

**4. Husband is About to Cheat.** This woman is unhappy because she suspects her significant other is contemplating infidelity or already scheming to cheat on her. Her motive is to make herself more attractive to win back his attention and affection and hopefully inspire him to stay faithful. Or move on!

**5. Husband is Cheating.** This woman is unhappy because her significant other is cheating! She hopes that a better body and/ or improved facial appearance will make him be faithful to her. Obviously, relationships are complicated, and rifts that trigger cheating may or may not be rooted in physical appearance. But a new body sure can get a cheating husband's attention long enough to help him realize what he's already got at home.

Meanwhile, all of the above categories provide an endless parade of soap-opera dramas that play out at my office/surgi-center/spa. Check this out: while a woman was getting butt implants, she left her cell phone with her husband, who was waiting in the lobby. Well, her ex-boyfriend texted while she was in surgery. All hell broke loose. A week after the procedure, the angry husband came to her follow-up appointment.

"Dr. Jeneby!" he shouted. "I want you to take those things out!"

"Hey," I said, "calm down. There are other patients in this office."

A week later, she came back to her two-week follow-up appointment with her husband's name tattooed across her neck! They're not together anymore. In fact, he came in a few weeks ago with somebody else, his third girlfriend getting surgery with me. He has married for the second time since then and brings *his first wife* to get procedures, too. What a country!

## Are You Listening? The Lost Art of Listening Can Make or Break Your Surgery

It's shocking how people have lost the ability to listen and follow instructions. This torments me and my staff every day, and we have to cancel 10 percent of procedures because they took a Motrin, Advil, or Anaprox the night before, in spite of having verbal, written, and video instructions not to.

*Whaaaat?*

The number one offense?

People don't read the written instructions that we give them. We provide *in writing* everything we've told them verbally multiple times!

"Do not take anything by mouth that can make you bleed," we repeat over and over. "There are about 50 to 100 things that can make you bleed. So, do not take Naproxen or Motrin IB, or any of the other things on this sheet."

They nod and accept the sheet of paper listing everything they are not supposed to take. The instructions are: "Only take Tylenol if you desperately need a pain reliever."

We also tell them not to take birth control pills for a week before surgery "because you could get a blood clot and it could kill you."

We spell it out in plain and simple language!

You'd think that would be a serious enough warning for someone to follow directions. Wrong.

Active listening is crucial for a patient to achieve the best outcome from their surgery. This has been taught to me by my malpractice carrier. They teach you to actively listen to a question, not just nod and wait until you can ask YOUR question.

"Now, can you understand what's going to happen to you?" I ask. "I'm going to cut here. I'm going to pull this up. I'm going to close it." Then I ask, "What did I just say?"

About 90 percent can't say what I just said. Maybe 10 percent can regurgitate. They're thinking about a text, groceries, job, Facebook, pets, or their kids. They're listening passively. *They're actively not listening.* I was taught to explain procedures and concepts at a sixth-grade reading level.

The illiteracy rate in San Antonio is 25 percent. Of those, 12.5 percent cannot read or write; the other 12.5 percent are functionally illiterate, meaning they have some ability to read and write, but not enough to function well in daily life or on a job. San Antonio is America's seventh largest city, has the second highest illiteracy rate among Texas cities, and ranks 67th out of 75 in comparably sized cities in the US.[4]

So, I do my spiel, but they interrupt with questions like: "When can I shower/have sex/go back to work/take a vacation/take off my bandages/exercise?"

I ask them to patiently let me round out my discussion and almost all their questions will be answered!

Sometimes I also face a barrier because I'm a Yankee doing business in Southern Texas. Sometimes they want me to spend an hour

---

4    https://www.mysapl.org/Portals/6/Files/About/StrategicPlan/CommunityProfile.pdf

discussing skin anatomy and every detail of what we're doing. I do an overview, and I have 10 to 30 minutes to answer questions, talk about risks, options, benefits, how much time they'll need off, and childcare.

When it comes to listening, I have four subsets of women who may or may not listen carefully. Upon first meeting, I'm constantly attempting to discern which category a woman fits into.

They are:

1. Highly intelligent. I should tell her everything.
2. Intelligent, but she nitpicks, so less is more. If I tell them everything, they will ask me 10,000 questions "just because."
3. Normal intelligence. I can tell her everything because she will listen and follow instructions.
4. Normal intelligence, but not well versed. I share as needed. We are the experts; she is in good hands and doesn't need to know every detail of what we're doing. Otherwise, it may scare her unnecessarily!

## Who's the Man (or Woman) Behind Your Makeover?

If you think I'm tough on screening women, I really zero in on the dynamics I observe between men and women when they come to a consult as a couple. I gotta deal with him/her too.

When the wife wants boobs and the husband is highly jealous, he sits there totally disinterested. Some guys even play on their phones.

I try to engage the significant other and try to get him to acknowledge that his wife is going to be off duty for a while.

"You know, she can't change the cat litter because that puts her at risk for infection. Will you be able to help out?"

Sometimes this draws a blank stare or downright annoyance.

But I have to warm him up to surgery because her successful outcome will depend on having help at home after the procedure.

Other times, it's easy. If surgery is the man's idea, he's like, "Oh yeah, I want her to go big! Big tits! When can she have this done? I'll do whatever, doc!"

When a man makes the appointment, he's like, "Oh that's my woman. She's doing this because I want her to have a nice rack."

On the other hand, when a woman initiates a breast aug, she wants to get her perkiness back because she had a baby or she's financially ready and now, they're sagging.

The ways that women finance surgery reveals a whole different drama. We had a young woman who was a stripper who brought in a gentleman in his 70s to pay for her surgery. He was walking with a cane!

*Ummm, paging Captain Obvious!*

Another patient had four different men pay for her surgery, and they all paid their "share" in cash. Stranger still, the husband picked her up every time. It seems he was in on the scam!

Observing all these dynamics is fascinating, and it's enabled me to categorize a subset of guys who participate in the procedures for their lovers, girlfriends, and wives. Here they are:

**Super Controlling Guys.** These guys are a-holes. They sit in the consult and do all the talking, while the woman just peeks over. When I ask her what she wants, she looks at him.

"You need to tell me what YOU want," I say. "Don't look at him. I'm going to be cutting on your body, so I need to hear from you."

**Great Guys.** They are pretty nice. They are loving husbands and boyfriends who, when the lady asks, "What do you think, honey?" they say, "Whatever you think is fine. I'm just here to support you."

**Jerks!** These guys are on the low end of significant others who accompany patients to consults. They are totally disengaged, playing video games on their phones, or looking totally unexcited to be here. Maybe they're insecure and fear that their beautified woman will attract a new guy and leave them.

The hardest couples that I deal with involve a smart woman with a controlling husband. She demands to know everything that I'm doing (over and above the "norm" for her procedure) and her husband talks to me like he's the doctor and knows more than what my Ivy League education, 18 years of experience, and board certification have instilled in me because he has done multiple "Google searches."

*There is no Dr. Google...* I say to myself.


## Male Patients Are a Whole Different Ball Game!

I stride into a consult with a new male patient. He's sitting calmly on the exam table, shakes my hand, looks me in the eye. His wife is sitting in a chair nearby.

"I got man boobs, Dr. Jeneby," he says. "Take care of it."

He doesn't look at his wife as if asking for permission with his eyes. He's ready to have surgery and doesn't ask anyone's consent. I always like to say the following at our meetings. Guys will let you operate on them in your garage if: One, the price is right. Two, they like you. They couldn't care less if your place has a rosy smell, or how the receptionist greeted them that day.

*Whew, sanity.*

Actually, about 95 percent of guys come alone; only about five percent arrive with a significant other.

Men—who only make up about 11 percent of our patients—generally make decisions easily and are simple to deal with.

I see about 20 men per month in my clinic.

If a guy likes his results, sometimes he doesn't come back. He just keeps steppin' with his new look and he's happy.

A big motivation for men to get plastic surgery—especially the increasingly popular procedures for hair implants and under-eye bag removal—is to look younger in order to compete with millennials in the workplace. Another motivation is that they're getting divorced and want to get back into the dating scene looking their best. Or they just started dating a younger chick and want to keep her attention.

Bottom line, money and sex are the biggest motivators for men who go under my surgical knife.

In contrast, women in their 50s and 60s prefer facelifts/brow-lifts/eyelifts to preserve as much of a youthful look as possible. I have had women truck drivers come in for facelift consults!

"Male patients are typically secretive," Anissa says. "They are less likely to want to be photographed or have their procedure broadcast live on Snapchat or Facebook. They are also acutely aware of the stigma of *not* looking beefy and brawny from working out if they are overweight or out of shape." Most just want to have nothing "bulging" through a tight-fitting T-shirt in the gym, among their friends or when going out.

*They don't like their "man tits" to be showing through a T-shirt!*

Liposuction is hugely popular with men on their love handles, man boobs, and abdomens. I call a surgery with man boobs and abdomen "Sparta" surgery. We try and make them look like the actors in the movie *300*. LOL. Some military men who want to pass their circumference test—a tape test that has maximum circumference of their waist in order to pass military "norms" as young as 19 years old—come in wanting lipo, but we tell them they'll be swollen for six or eight weeks.

Another big draw: penis enlargement. The procedure costs $25,000 and involves expanding the girth by implanting fat from another part of the body. A lot of guys who come in for a penis enlargement consultation simply want confirmation that their penis is average size, not small. Turns out, their wife or girlfriend has been pressuring them to seek a larger size. *That sucks.*

## One Man's Cosmetic Procedure Provides a New Outlook on Life

When David L. hit his late 30s, he felt so self-conscious about his eye bags, he didn't want to leave the house. This puffiness under his eyes made him look old and tired. Unfortunately, the genetic cards were stacked against him, because his mother and his uncle were both plagued by under-eye bags that only got worse with age.

"At first," David said during an interview for this book, "it was a little nuisance. Then it became more of something that made me want to go out less and less in public. I felt like, 'There's really nothing I can do about it.' It looked bad from all angles."

David confided in his wife that he was unhappy with his appearance.

"We've always had a good, solid marriage," he said, "but I've always complained to my wife about my eye bags." At the same time, he was impressed that she was reversing the aging process by using various facial treatments. He was also ambitious in his education and career. David wanted to look and feel his best for his wife and for his work in nursing and physical therapy—two professions that require a lot of face-to-face time with patients and people in general.

"I was in school to become a nurse practitioner," David recalled. "I had finished a degree in physical therapy and transitioned from an old job, and I was looking for work in a therapy field."

Then David began to fear that the age-adding under-eye bags were blocking his ability to find employment in his area of expertise.

"I had a hard time getting hired," David recalled. "I had really good academic credentials. Good experience. Military background."

Then it hit him: "I came to the personal conclusion that maybe I didn't look good enough or I looked too old because of the bags. They make you look old and tired, even if you don't feel old and tired. I thought, 'Maybe I'm not appealing enough. Maybe I'm too old.' Appearing too old to potential employers prompted me to take action."

David refused to hide away in shame and unemployment. So, he started searching for solutions. First, he watched YouTube videos by people who had undergone a surgical procedure to remove their under-eye bags.

"It looked pretty good," he said. "After I looked at the videos, I decided, 'One day, I'm going to get this.'"

Then he did an online search for Plastic Surgeons who perform the procedure, which is called blepharoplasty.

"Dr. Jeneby's website popped up first," David said. "I thought, 'It seems like he's got a lot of credentials… and I don't see anything negative about him.' So, I scheduled an appointment. I was nervous. Anytime you have surgery, there's a chance a minor thing can go wrong."

When we met for the first time at his consultation, David said I wasn't like a typical surgeon because I greeted him by saying, "Hey, bro, how's it going?"

My demeanor made him feel like he was talking with a friend.

"My first impression of Dr. Jeneby was that he seemed more of a regular guy than a lot of doctors, who can be too clinical," he said. "Usually a physician doesn't say, 'Hey, man, check this out.' He's always relaxed and always has a smile."

David said he also trusted me because of my credentials, which he knew required significant hard work and skill to achieve. He respected that I was board certified and Joint Commission certified.

"Not everybody can do that," he said, "especially in cosmetic surgery, which is above and beyond your regular course of study. That's pretty rigorous."

Another thing David appreciated was having the ability to read through positive reviews online from my satisfied patients. That sealed the deal for him: he knew he'd found the perfect place to rid him of his eye-bag problem.

"Unlike internal surgery where nobody can see the final product," David said, "with plastic surgery, it's out there for the whole world to see. It's an advertisement. If you do it wrong, people will know."

David did not contact any other Plastic Surgeons.

"Dr. Jeneby was the first name I saw, and he had such good recommendations, I said, 'I think I'm going to go here, especially since he's so prominent in Texas.' I liked that he was a fellow Texan."

So, David, who had saved money every month to have this procedure someday, paid $4,000 out of pocket. That included preliminary eye exams with an eye specialist prior to surgery, as well as a year of follow-up after the procedure.

"I was ready to get it done and I didn't feel any stigma or reservations about it," he said. "I was counting down the time to surgery."

In November of 2017, it was game time.

"They started the IV in the pre-op room, and Dr. Jeneby talked to me. After pre-op, they walked me into the surgical suite. I remember lying on the table, and the nurse began the loading dose."

"Count backward from ten," she said.

"Ten...nine..."

David was amazed: "The next thing I knew, I was waking up after surgery. I felt great post-surgery. My wife was surprised."

His eyes were bandaged, so his wife helped him dress.

"Do you feel nauseous or any pain?" the staff asked him.

"No, actually I feel hungry," David said, because he hadn't eaten dinner the night before to prepare for surgery. "No nausea at all."

"Any pain?"

"No."

David's wife took him out for a chocolate shake, which he finished and still felt fine.

"I didn't feel any pain or discomfort, just swelling," he said. "Dr. Jeneby sent me home with mild narcotics, a stool softener, and nighttime medication, which was a sleeping aid and pain reliever. I didn't have to take anything. I did elevating and icing and didn't have complications."

He removed the eye patches when they left the clinic, but the sutures remained in place.

"It's kind of weird," David said. "You have all this bruising and stitches hanging off your face. It looks horrific, but it didn't hurt. The swelling receded, and Dr. Jeneby snipped and pulled out the stitches."

Next came an exercise in patience.

"The lesson I learned was being patient for the final results to kick in," David said. "I still saw some bagginess in my perception. Part of the recovery regimen was to use strips of sticky paper called Steri-Strips as a physiological crutch with cold packs. I did that religiously. I felt I was in that interim state."

David was worried about a condition called ectropion, where the lower eyelids pull down and punch out, exposing the inner eyelid.

"The healing naturally wants to tighten up," he said. "I religiously did the massage and taping, and Dr. Jeneby said I did well on that aspect, because sometimes people get lazy with their post-surgery regimen."

Still, David was worried that the surgery was not successful.

"A couple times, I questioned Dr. Jeneby," David said. "I was saying, 'I don't know if I was a good candidate for this. I don't know if it was worth it.' He continually reassured me that everything was okay, telling me that the skin under the eyes is tough tissue to heal. He explained that it's unique among the skin tissue because it's really thin and fragile, and that I just needed to be patient. Dr. Jeneby showed a remarkable degree of patience with me and my questions. He even offered to let me talk to other individuals who'd had the surgery. I didn't want to intrude on them and complain."

To accelerate the process, David had two post-surgical laser treatments that showed results.

"Then it finally kicked in," David said. "The main judgement came from my wife. She's very no-nonsense and will tell me the straight-up truth. She doesn't sugar coat. One day, she said, 'Wow, you look really good!'"

Shortly after that, David came in for a check-up.

"You look really good," said Nancy, our aesthetician.

Compliments from his wife and Nancy helped David see that he really did look better.

"We're always going to be our worst own critic," he said.

So, did the now-younger-looking David finally get the job?

"After nurse practitioner school," he said, "I lost my desire to work in the health care field."

He totally shifted gears and started his own small business. Now he's running a store, interacting with the public, and feeling great about it.

So how does he feel now?

"Having my eye bags done makes my face look younger," he said. "The rest of me feels younger. I feel like going out more in public. I don't feel like I have to shorten the time I spend in public or curtail going out. You can't stay home under a rock."

Besides boosting his confidence, the cosmetic procedure invigorated his interest in ways to promote youthfulness.

"I've always been interested in anti-aging stuff," he said. "The eye-bag procedure was a good stepping stone. I started looking at other lifestyle changes—exercise, diet, medical practices that physicians tell patients, such as cholesterol and saturated fats."

He also observed the struggles that his mother was having on a certain medication that the family had not researched to know the risks and side effects.

So, David began a quest to learn as much as possible about how to stay healthy and youthful through his lifestyle. He began incorporating organic foods, water filters, shower head filters, air cleaners and scrubbers, and rigorous calisthenics and body weight training that he incorporates throughout the day.

"I've made continuous little discoveries here," he said. "Having my eye bags removed created a good snowball effect. It opened up my thinking on the anti-aging, life extension process. Unfortunately, we never learned this information in school, so you have to go above and beyond to learn it yourself. I don't want to end up looking at all old."

David is now 50.

"Not to sound conceited," he said, "but I get a lot of compliments. People usually guess my age around 30. That feels good."

In fact, he has become so physically fit that strangers comment, "Dude, you look like Wolverine!" They're referring to Hugh Jackman, the actor who has great muscle definition and is very fit in the *X-Men* films.

David says his success with surgery has inspired his wife to consider cosmetic procedures as well.

So, did David fear a stigma about men getting plastic surgery?

"I don't think it's such a stigma anymore," he said. "You see actors and actresses getting it done. It's obvious they've had something done. The techniques have advanced. The safeties have advanced. The frequencies and qualities have advanced. I don't think most people would find a stigma associated with it. It's more of a stigma to remain looking old. Employers want to hire younger people; they can pay them less and they may believe a younger person is sick less often. I hear lots of stories of people getting procedures done to remain competitive in their job."

And what's David's recommendation to other men who are considering plastic surgery to look and feel better?

"With any procedure, there's a risk. So, take a smart, calculated, well thought-out risk. I researched Dr. Jeneby. I knew my own health was good."

Now he's looking and feeling so great, his advice is very strong: "I would say have it done."


## Everyone Wants to Date the Doctor

When you appear on billboards, national TV programs, high-profile radio shows, as well as in local and national magazines, you tend to develop a fan club. Even better, my patients are walking, talking advertisements for the excellent work that I do.

As a result, all of this adds up to "local celebrity" status in San Antonio. I have a *ball* with it when people recognize me in restaurants and at events and are super nice and accommodating as a result. At first, I was a little embarrassed, but I kind of just settled into it!

One crazy result, however, is that my staff encounters some female patients who are gaga over the doc.

"In some cases, patients are just here to get a glimpse of him," Anissa says with a laugh. "They're enamored by him. They ask me, 'Is his hair real? Have you ever touched it? Have you ever brushed it?' Young and old women ask really odd questions. They see him on billboards or on TV on *Dancing with the Stars*. He was on the local edition, so they thought he was on the national show. He's also been on *Inside Edition* several times. This is San Antonio. It's not like New York where they have TV stars all over. So, he's risen to this celebrity status that makes some women swoon."

Anissa adds, "When I first started, I was not used to it. I'd tell the patient in the exam room, 'Dr. Jeneby will be in here shortly.' I'd give them a garment, but I'd come back into the room—and they'd be completely naked! So, I always tell Dr. Jeneby before we enter, 'She may or may not be naked.' If they are naked, we make them put on a garment. I've also had women laying seductively on the exam table when we walk in. They're in for a breast aug, so obviously they have to expose their breasts, but they're all laid out in a seductive pose."

We require patients to behave appropriately.

"Please sit up so I can measure your breasts," Anissa tells them. "Dr. Jeneby realizes what they're doing. The women stumble over their words. They say things like, 'Oh my God, I can't believe I'm meeting you! I'm so embarrassed! My breasts aren't perfect. You probably look at perfect breasts all day.'"

Anissa shows no reaction: "I've learned to flat-face it. We're here to provide a professional service, so we keep everything strictly business."

As such, my clinic is a No-Drama Zone for women who have dated me or who have wanted to date me. Now that I'm extremely happily married, this is a thing of the past and was hilarious. But my trusted clinical manager Sylvia Montes, who has worked for me for 14 years, is like a Doberman Pinscher protecting the castle that Dr. Jeneby built. Nobody can get past her!

"He didn't want girlfriends coming here if he wasn't 100 percent serious with them," she says. "He had strict boundaries to make sure we keep the office, surgery center and spa a drama-free zone. When he'd start dating someone, he'd tell her, 'The office is off limits. You can't just show up or drop by.' I was his bodyguard to keep them from 'rolling up in here,' trying to get free Botox."

Sometimes this required Sylvia to go above and beyond the call of duty to shield me from obsessed fans.

"One in particular was psycho-crazy," Sylvia recalls. "We were having a surprise birthday party for him, and she called the office and we talked after hours on my cell phone. A big mistake! Every day after they broke up, she'd call me in my car at 5:00 p.m. and say, 'Is he seeing someone else?' I told her, 'My loyalty is to him, not to you.' Then I told him, 'You need to talk to this chick! She needs to stop calling me.' I had to block her number. That's how crazy she was. He told her, 'Stop bothering my staff with this nonsense!'"

## Do New Boobs Boost Self-Esteem and Self-image?

So, do new boobs boost self-esteem? And is it okay that a person gains confidence from an external characteristic?

*Hell, yeah!*

"I had very low self-esteem," says Anissa, who got boobs for herself, not her fiancé. "It certainly has enhanced my private life, but I did this for me. A partner can come and go, but these boobs are mine forever. I did it for me."

Anissa says a lot of patients confide their biggest fears and dreams in the process of improving the look of their bodies. "This is more than just a Plastic Surgeon's office. I've had so many patients cry to me at a consultation. They break down and start crying because they haven't told anybody how badly they feel. It feels good to them that they have somebody to talk to."

After a procedure, we offer a year's worth of follow-ups, so we maintain a strong relationship with each patient. This enables us to observe how altering one's body really can improve their quality of life on many levels.

"The outside changes can precipitate an inside change," Anissa says. "Once they get up and can look in the mirror and say, 'I like or I love what I see,' it starts to reprogram their mind with a whole new train of thought. It changes their negative self-talk and criticism about saggy boobs into something positive, and they start to radiate that excitement from the inside out. The world responds accordingly when they interact with people in a more upbeat manner."

It's so exciting and fulfilling for us to witness someone really blossom when they finally feel good about themselves after feeling down for so long.

We help people get their lives back, and what more thrilling way can you possibly spend your day? I love transforming people's lives for the better. It's like being a magician, and my scalpel is a magic wand, helping me sculpt bodies into something more beautiful.

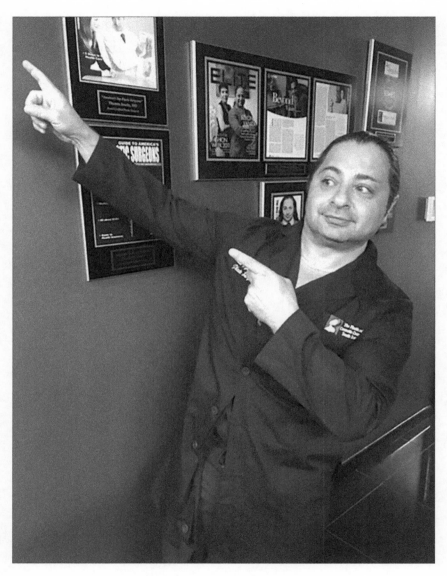

Before entering the OR jungle!

# 2
# Shocking Scenes from the OR and Beyond

*"I don't go crazy.*
*I am crazy.*
*I just go normal from time to time."*

—*Unknown*

It's six in the morning, and I'm jabbing a silver metal tube throughout my patient's subcutaneous abdomen as she lies unconscious on the operating table. Surrounded by my extraordinary OR team in my private operating room, I couldn't be happier. This is my sanctuary away from the world. For the next five hours, I will be focusing on sculpting this woman into a new and improved version of herself.

We're doing a mega makeover: Brazilian Butt Lift, breast aug, tummy tuck, and liposuction. All at once!

"Dr. Jeneby," says my social media maestro Ana, aiming a video camera at me, "Say hi to everybody watching live on Snapchat!"

"Hey, guys, what's up?" I say while my arm gets a super workout, pushing the long, metal wand in and out of my patient's large belly that jiggles with every stroke. "This is a long procedure. Right now, I'm injecting fluid through the belly button area, because we're starting her off with lipo."

I've already drawn purple lines all over her stomach. White tape covers her nipples. Her torso is the only thing exposed in the entire OR, which is draped with sterile blue paper.

"We're about to harvest the fat from her abdomen, her lower back, and her upper back," I say, "then later we'll inject the fat into her butt for a BBL."

I'm wearing black scrubs covered by a blue surgical gown, white latex gloves, and a custom-made black skull cap embroidered with DR. JENEBY PLASTIC SURGERY. My safety glasses have a spot-light attached with magnifying loupes, so the light shines directly on what I'm doing.

"This is the biggest procedure that we do," I add. "It includes Lipo 360, a BBL, a breast aug, and a tummy tuck! Full super Mommy Makeover!"

The camera shows a sign listing the procedures we offer and the number to text to ask a question or make an appointment.

"If you have questions or want more information about our procedures," Ana says, "just text MOMMY to 38470 and tell us what you want." Ana focuses the camera on a sign taped to the wall that lists: Boobs, Butt, Hot, Lipo, Mommy, Tummy. Then she tells me:

"Dr. Jeneby, Quintero B. texted and said, 'Hi, I want this so bad, but I'm so nervous!'"

"I'll be awesome!" I exclaim. "Don't worry about it. You've got my awesome plastic surgery team that's been together for five years.

We've had people on multiple medications and our anesthesiologist can make sure you're safe. You have nothing to worry about. It will be awesome!"

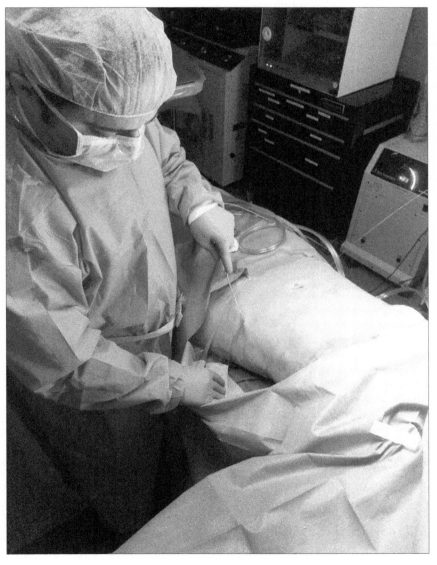

Doin' lipo—I'm in my zone!

I glance down at my hand, continuously ramming our patient's subcutaneous abdomen, and I say, "Right now I'm injecting a warm saline solution mixed with lidocaine and epinephrine. That will keep her warm and reduce the swelling and pain. This fluid will help break up the fat and control bleeding. Lipo is traumatic, so this will help keep her comfortable."

Hip-hop music booms in the background, along with the beeping of monitors that my anesthesiologist, Dr. Flores, is watching, along with the patient's vitals to make sure she's stable and healthy throughout the procedure. Having my own Joint Commission accredited private surgery center and an anesthesiologist on hand ensures that everything we do protects our patient's safety as the top priority.

"We're keeping everything as safe as possible," I say. "Dr. Flores is giving her beautiful anesthetic as usual. She is a very accomplished anesthesiologist."

Ana smiles. "Dr. Jeneby, we're getting lots of questions. We love our San Antonio peeps! Someone is asking, 'Does your liposuction tube go into the intestines?'"

"No," I say over a buzzing sound, looking at the camera, "this device does not go in the intestines. We're on top of the body, which is fascia. Think of the body like a big, long sausage. You have the casing over the pepperoni. I'm trained to stay above that casing. That's my field. That's why surgical procedures like this will never be automated in my lifetime."

I do surgeries live on social media, so I can demystify the process and show what really happens. That way, people know exactly how it works, and they see that I'm a forever student of plastic surgery, so they can trust me to perform procedures that will change their lives for the better. Live social media is the best marketing tool ever, because it allows people to get to know me and watch my meticulous attention to detail in a surprisingly fun, high-energy environment. Plus, I love taking viewers' questions. What started out as a marketing tool has turned into an information spigot which makes the patients feel more at ease with me.

"We also stay really safe by giving a blood thinner. We'll watch her overnight in our hotel suite with an RN," I add as blood drips over the purple lines I have drawn across her abdomen to delineate where to cut for her tummy tuck.

"We're gonna make this girl look significantly more contoured," I say. "This woman is 5'2" and weighs 220 pounds. This is not a weight-loss procedure. This is a contouring procedure. And she has to follow a weight-loss plan as part of the recovery process."

Ana says, "One of our live viewers is texting, 'Oh my goodness, this woman is so brave. She's going to be in so much pain. You go, girl!'"

Hearts flash across Ana's phone screen as people text questions. She says, "Dr. Jeneby, someone in Austin is texting, 'Does it hurt?'"

"Good question," I say, facing the camera and steadily moving the lipo wand in and out. "This is the best arm workout ever! To answer your question about pain, since she's having work done in the front and in the back, she'll have to lie on her side for two weeks, but she can get back to exercising in three to four weeks. So yes, there is pain, but we'll give her medication, we'll monitor her overnight in a private hotel suite with a nurse, and she'll go home with meds to keep her comfortable."

A short time later, I use the same wand to extract the fat that's loosened up by the warm liquid and the stabbing motion that I make throughout her belly button. "Now I'm harvesting the fat."

Thick, pink goo surges through a clear tube connected to my wand, and it spirals around the tube on a tray over the patient, who's draped in sterile blue cloth like everything else in the OR. "I'm suctioning the fat. See how it's collecting in that container?"

Ana aims the camera so hundreds, if not thousands, of our viewers anywhere in the world can watch this procedure. I am amazed that viewers from England, New Zealand, the Philippines, Ukraine, Sweden, and 20 other countries are watching!

I glance at the clear container that's filling up with pink fat.

"See this beautiful fat harvesting in there?" I say, glancing at the camera. "All this fat is going to be placed in her buttocks area."

I gaze at the fat. "This is beautiful, bright yellow fat. It's pink because some blood has mixed in. It's like a blood-orange martini."

"Or a strawberry-banana smoothie," says my longtime ace surgical technician, Britany. She and I have been working together for years. When she started, she was super quiet, but just like Dr. Frankenstein's monster, now she speaks her mind and handles her business in the OR like a boss! She says, "It's all your fault—you made me this way!" Right!

"I am so fortunate to have my pro team in the OR," I say, as two other techs keep all the equipment in order and ready for the next steps.

"Next we're going to turn her over," I say, holding up a glass vial of thick, pink liquid. "We got this from the upper abdomen. Beautiful, bright, yellow fat. We like to see that. Not red, yellow."

I resume the lipo that loosens the fat and enables me to suction it out as her belly shakes. Meanwhile, Britany looks like she's about to bake a cake. Using giant plastic syringes that look like frosting tubes used for decorating cakes, she's injecting the pink liquid fat into two round strainers with handles. Those strainers are secured over what look like two silver metal cake pans, and the fat is dripping down through the strainers into the pans. It literally looks like strawberry cake batter.

But it's fat that will be injected into this woman's backside to give her a beautiful contour for a Brazilian Butt Lift.

"This way we don't have to use implants," I say. "We're using her own fat."

Britany uses a spatula-like instrument to stir the fat in the strainer. "I'm sifting through the fat right now," she says. "We're using syringes, so we can transfer it into the butt."

I point to the woman's upper abdomen where I just lipo'd out fat. "You can see that it's already flatter," I say.

Next, the patient is turned over, and I move the lipo wand into her upper back, then her lower back.

"I'm injecting the fluid to loosen the fat," I say. "There's no need for a hospital stay, because we didn't take more than five liters of fat."

I point to her butt, which is covered in iodine-soaked plastic wrap. "We'll add a little bit more to the left butt because it's slightly smaller. We're going to curve in her waist, pinch it in, to create a nice hourglass shape."

Meanwhile, Britany is pouring more fat through the strainers and it's dripping into the pans. "We have to get it down to the good fat, then put it into one of these syringes."

"We're actually working on 10 areas of her body," I add.

Finally, it's time for the injection.

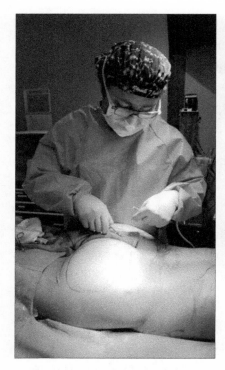

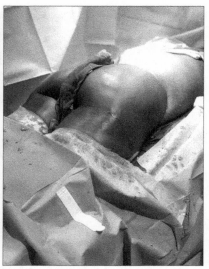

It IS all about the bass!

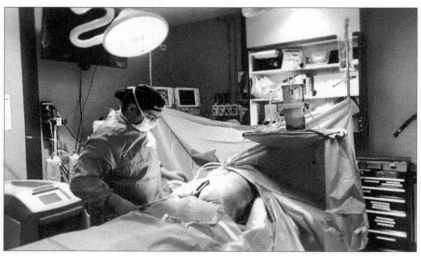

"Here comes the fat!" I announce as I inject a needle into her left buttock. It's attached to a giant plastic syringe full of the pink fat. I execute the butt injection using the same back-and-forth jamming motion that I used for lipo. We now use a closed-loop lipo and fat grafting machine that the girls never have to sift through or touch! It makes the procedure much more efficient and does not manipulate the already traumatized fat!

"You can start to see that this is pulling up," I say as I point to a nice curve that's forming on her left buttock and creating definition at the base of her back.

"Hey, guys on Snapchat, we're at 210 cc's," I say as I continuously ram the needle into her increasingly rounder butt to evenly distribute the injection of fat. "You can see the difference now." I peel away the plastic from her right buttock, which is now much smaller. "When we remove this, you can see the dramatic difference."

Next, I'm standing on the other side of the operating table, beside her right buttock, which sits lower and flatter than the now plumped-up, rounded left buttock.

"At this level, you can see the height of this," I say. "It's another centimeter projecting upward. She can run in about two weeks and exercise fully in about three weeks."

Now I'm injecting the fat with a ramming motion through a hole on the right side of the buttock. After that, I stitch up the injection holes on each side.

"Dr. Jeneby," Ana says, "A viewer is asking, 'What if I want to go bigger after the procedure?'"

I answer, "If you want to go bigger after the procedure, you have to gain weight or add an implant. You can use fat or implants.

Fat is nature's own implant. Because it's living. You're putting it back into an area and hope that it lives. Fat requires blood supply."

We wrap up the BBL, and I say, "There's the BootyMatic 1000!"

Then we flip the patient to start on her boob job. As I use a scalpel to open the flesh below her right breast, I say, "We've already contoured her buttocks. We did almost four liters of lipo and injected about 1,000 cc's into each butt cheek! Then we turned her over for the adjustable implant procedure."

The breast aug involves making a 1.5-inch incision at the bottom of each breast, then using a laser-type device called a Bovie that simultaneously cuts and cauterizes the skin and fat. Smoke or steam literally rise from the incision that has very little bleeding. Then we irrigate the area under the pectoralis muscle with fluid to flush out any potential bacteria and reduce the risk of infection. I sew in a one-inch plastic port that will be attached to the adjustable implant pouch. I do this by nestling the port into the fat, which looks like pinkish-yellow pomegranate seeds held open by a tiny fork.

Then I insert the rolled-up pouch, which is soaked in iodine as a disinfectant. Britany helps me inject saline through the port into the implant, which expands to the size of as many cc's as we need to meet the patient's cup size request.

For example, she may go up to a 36C, but ultimately can be a D by coming back in a few months for us to inject more saline into the adjustable implant. The gradual expansion is far less painful than waking up with giant implants that have suddenly stretched the skin and muscle.

As we perform this procedure, I chat with my staff about the importance of living your dreams.

"For a lot of people, having surgery is their dream," I say. "It's your time now. Live a little! A lot of my friends who are doctors die early in their fifties after doing all this hard work!"

"Don't be a Debbie Downer," says Britany, a quintessential millennial.

"I'm just saying, live a little," I add over suction sounds. "They never get a chance to get their butt fixed. And who doesn't like a nice butt?"

After seamlessly stitching up her breast incisions, I announce, "Now we're going to the abdomen. Time for the tummy tuck!"

I'm on one side of her; Britany is on the other side. I've drawn a purple line across her abdomen, just below the round ridge of fat between her belly button and her groin. I draw vertical lines.

I take my scalpel and cut the skin straight across the purple line.

"Okay, I'm going to start," I announce as a Prince song plays.

Then I use the Bovie to slice through the fat. The abdomen becomes loose and jiggly as I hold it down with my left hand and cut with my right hand.

Steam rises from the cut. I'm cutting deeply through layers of pink-speckled, yellow abdominal fat.

"We have teamwork!" I say.

"Thanks for the sandwiches today," Britany says.

"You earned it!"

Now, I'm peeling back the roll of lower abdominal fat, which Britany holds back. Then I cut off pieces of skin.

"Look at that wedge!" Britany says, holding up what looks like a giant piece of pie, but it's really skin over a few inches of fat. We measure it. Its removal leaves a triangular flap hanging down on the right side of the patient's abdomen.

Now Sheila E. is playing.

"This is like tailoring the skin," I say playfully.

We've created a fishtail-shaped flap of skin that's a few inches thick with skin and fat. I'm slicing out more fat.

"Someone asked what the BMI is for this surgery," Ana says.

"High 30s, low 40s," I say. "She's surprisingly healthy because she's young. If you don't have the health, you can't do this. You have to get medical clearances. And don't hold back anything from me, like smoking. Because I'll find out. I do drug tests. Our anesthesiologist has to know what you're taking." I slice off another giant pie-shaped slice of skin and fat.

"Alright, let's mark her up," I say. "Everything looks good. We're going to get her ready to close."

As the camera focuses on a white bowl full of triangle-shaped skin and fat that looks like apple pie, I'm suctioning the open abdomen, which is literally sliced open from hip to hip. I cut loose, jagged skin along the edge of the abdominal incision, then I cauterize it. Next, I'm stitching up beneath the abdominal flap as Britany holds it open. It's inside out, splayed open and upward, and it looks like two lungs.

Next, I make her a new belly button that's smaller and prettier. *People are very specific about their belly buttons. Don't F this up!*

Then I slice off the triangular flaps and sew in drainage tubes on the right and left sides. "We're doing some last-minute nips and tucks and cutting," I say, cutting something over the right hip. "This is a dog ear. It's wrapped around. We're going to continue this incision," I say while slicing. "See, that lays out like this. It's called a dog ear, and it comes right off like a little dog ear, see? So, I'm just going to lipo the dog ear here to make a smooth transition," I say while ramming the lipo stick into her abdomen. "See how flat that lies? That's why Plastic Surgeons get paid! We're dog ear masters!"

I compliment my team, including the anesthesiologist. "You've done a kick-ass job this whole case, keeping this lovely lady comfortable." Then I tell our viewers, "You have to go with the best plastic and the best anesthesia. These procedures aren't dangerous in themselves. Just make sure your anesthesia team is top notch. We have the best in the city."

I look down at all that we've done over the past five hours. I feel exhilarated because I get to do what I love every day and change people's lives for the better.

"Her body has changed significantly, as much as you could ever think it would," I say. "She's going to have to do her own dieting and weight loss. She's agreed to that to finish her transformation."

What a day!

## Butt Lift Gone Bad

After surgery, it's time for consults. I head into the first patient's room. I'm greeted by a man and a woman who barely speak English. Turns out, she had a substance injected into her lips and into her butt in Mexico. She doesn't know what it is and does not remember who did it!

"What's in her butt?" I ask. "What's in her lips?"

They don't know. Her butt is *purple* from the inflammation of the whatever is inside her. *Purple!*

*What the f@#%!*

It may have been motor oil or industrial-grade silicone, like the stuff in commercial glue or motor lubricant!

"I can't fix that," I say. "I'd have to completely cut off your lips from inside your mouth, and you'd have no lips."

This woman was straight off one of those TV shows about botched plastic surgeries.

The bottom line is this: if you're going to have surgery, do it in the United States with a reputable, board-certified surgeon who has a proven track record of success. Or if you are having a procedure in another country, check their credentials to ensure that he or she is an authentic, board-certified Plastic Surgeon in that country.

## NeoGraft Hair Transplant on Billy Madison

That afternoon, I perform an increasingly popular procedure for men and women who are experiencing hair loss. It's called NeoGraft and it involves taking a live hair follicle from one part of the body and implanting it in the place where you want hair to grow.

My patient on this day is radio superstar Billy Madison of *The Billy Madison Show*, "a funny, irreverent show built for guys," according to http://www.unitedstations.com/Show/Index/1066. The now-nationally syndicated morning show started on 99.5 KISS-FM in San Antonio in 2011.

We bring Billy into Spa Black, where he's slightly sedated and numbed across the forehead and back of his head. One of my staff members uses a little machine that clicks holes over the hair follicle to both harvest the healthy one from the back of his head, then implant it at his front hairline.

"This is awesome," he says. "This is phenomenal. You don't feel anything. No scars. I can't wait to see it. Dude, this is awesome, like

I didn't know what to expect, but I didn't feel any pain. NeoGraft is the way to go."

He smiles. "They take little hairs from the back of your head and put them on the top of your head. That's it. Then you look fantastic! It's as simple as that. The hair on the back doesn't die. Dr. J. is making men hot again!"

"You're such a good patient, man," I say. "It's a Billy Makeover."


## Man Boobs and Love Handles Be Gone!

Next, I dash back into the OR where I perform another popular procedure for men: liposuction on the man boob.

"We're broadcasting live on Facebook and Snapchat," I say as my lipo wand moves back and forth inside the man's breast fat. He's sedated, and my anesthesiologist is monitoring his vitals and medications. "Thanks for joining us."

His nipple is taped for broadcast, and we joke about exposing it.

"Free the nipple!" Britany says.

"You can see the difference here," I say, pointing to the reduced size of the first breast compared to the one that remains to be done.

"Flat," I say, touching the left lipo'd breast. Then I touch the bigger one and say, "Full." I am glowing with satisfaction.

Next, I insert a needle with a lighted red tip glowing through the skin of the breast as I move it slowly around the tissue.

Someone on social media asks, "Does this cause ultra-sensitivity to the nipple?"

"Good question," I say. "It can. But usually not. See, the skin is shrinking. It's really an awesome, awesome tool."

I point to the breast. "Normally I would open this up under the nipple and remove the rest of the breast tissue. But he doesn't really need that. And if he does have more breast tissue, we won't know for a year. I can take that out."

Another popular procedure for men (and women) to remove love handles is CoolSculpting, which literally freezes the fat and allows it to get flushed out by the body naturally. It's an alternative to surgery in some cases. We can do all that!

## Vaginal Rejuvenation Triggers Dirty Mind

Our Spa Black provides a service called Vaginal Rejuvenation, which is essentially tightening inside and/or outside. A lot of women who've had children say this procedure can greatly enhance their sex lives for both themselves and their partners.

Well, one day a controlling man brought his wife in, and Britany was performing the procedure behind a curtain separating the woman from her husband. Typically, the husband waits in the lobby, but this guy insisted on being in there.

After Britany inserted the tube inside the woman's vagina to do the procedure, the man asked, "Is that turning her on?"

Britany was unsure if he was asking about herself or his wife. And she didn't want to know.

"Sir, you need to vacate the area," she said.

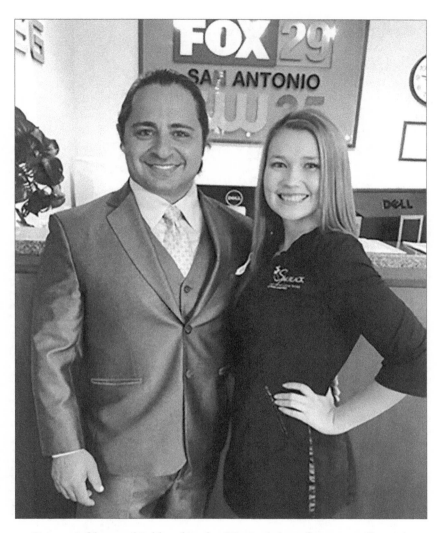

Britany is like my third hand in the OR. And she is fluent in millennial.

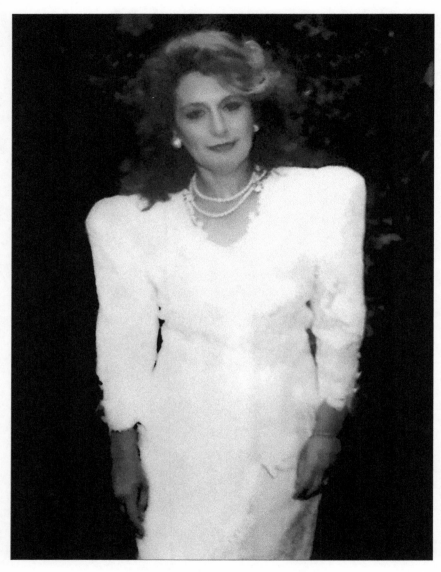

My mom: beauty, brains, and all business!

# 3
# My Family's Story

*"Remember,*
*as far as everyone knows,*
*we are a nice normal family."*

—*Unknown*

## Dr. Lamya Alarif aka Mom

My parents were from the Southwestern part of Turkey, so we're mostly Kurdish. My mother's father, my grandfather, was a diplomat and sent her to the US for school when she was 14. She had her first degree, a Bachelor of Science in biology, by 16. By 19, she had a master's in biology from Georgetown University, where she was offered a scholarship to stay and pursue graduate work towards a PhD in molecular biology.

*My mom is the smart one of the fam.*

She started but had to interrupt her studies to return home and marry my father in a prearranged marriage. My father was finishing his OB/GYN studies. I was born, followed by my sister a year later.

How do we get from there to here? I guess you could blame it on my diarrhea, hyperbilirubinemia, and jaundice. My mother was scared that something was gravely wrong with me. She was concerned that if I developed major problems, that I was going to have serious, lifelong medical issues.

She knew the care I could get in the US was the best in the world, and she would not have to worry about my diarrhea. She also knew the education we'd receive would be number one.

"I'm leaving," she told my father. She boldly took my sister and me—with just $400 in her pocket!—back to Washington, DC, where she knew I could get the best treatment. She tackled this challenge with incredible courage, strength, and risk, because now she was a single mom in the US. What balls!

My health issue resolved itself quickly.

Today, Mom recalls, "I was scared for him when he was young. I knew in the US he could get vaccines and see American-trained pediatricians."

Nutrition and care were my cure, thankfully, and that freed her to restart her PhD—this time with two little kids crawling all over her papers.

We lived with Uncle Abdullah Alarif, the sweetest uncle ever, who took care of us. Our grandmother, Bibi, who didn't know any English, came over after a year and helped Mom. Bibi was a super-kind woman with really thick, calloused feet.

We were this little family with one mom, an uncle, and a grand-mother, all living in a small house. All I knew was happiness. We entertained ourselves by playing outside, and we had a ball. We didn't have a lot of money. No iPhones, iPads, or video games.

We didn't even have enough money for a Big Wheel; we had to

share one with a friend. We were just scraping by; spending money on clothes was not a priority for our mom.

As a result, my sister Resha and I wore cheap clothes, such as low-budget Toughskins jeans while other kids were wearing pricier Levi's.

"Look at Tayf with the Toughskin jeans!" one girl from a prominent family taunted with her sing-songy voice. I felt terrible!

Once people started making fun of my clothes—while they were wearing Izods and polos and high-end clothes, I thought, "Someday I'm gonna blow it out and have everything I want, so no one ever talks to me like this again!"

It was a big problem, and it triggered me to dream big. I mean, I was nine years old, wishing for a Lamborghini. So, I listened to my mom about how education would lay the foundation for a good life, and nothing was going to distract me from making it big someday.

## Dad, the OB/GYN, Arrives

When our father came over to the US after he finished his schooling, we moved into our own house. That's when he gave me something that I cherish to this day: a genuine, old-school black doctor's bag with a real stethoscope.

It was no secret that for as long as I can remember, I've wanted to be a doctor. Having "Dr." before my name seemed pre-programmed in my genetics, because medical degrees and doctorates are embedded in my family's DNA. Besides my dad being a doctor, his father was an OB/GYN. Plus, we have a huge number of MDs and PhDs in our extended family on both my parents' sides.

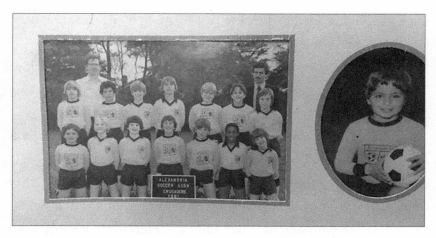

**Me as a young soccer stud.**

My grandfather, Ismail Alarif, PhD, was a diplomat. He'd been involved in the 1950s revolution to free Iraq from the Brits. He was second in command in the country.

So, with all this family history, I announced as a kid: "I'm going to be a doctor."

"Of course, you are," my sister, Resha, remembers, adding that it was never an option or a question.

Meanwhile, as we grew up, our father was busy being an OB/GYN all the time. He was always delivering babies.

On Sundays, though, he would pack us up and drive to southern Maryland where he worked. He took us into his office where he did follow-up patient care and rounds. We were exposed to hospitals, so nothing was intimidating.

Curiously, the gender ratio in his workplace tended to be similar to my current situation! He was the only guy, and the rest of the people he was surrounded by, nurses and patients included, were all women. I was pretty precocious, and the nurses loved me. I'd sit at the nurse's station and solve my Rubik's Cube over and over.

I don't know if there's some strange coincidence between those early years of being surrounded by all women while at "work," and my practice now, but the ratio is the same: I'm the only guy surrounded by all these women in my practice! *Yikes.*

At the end of the Sunday workday, our dad would cap the day off with a trip to McDonald's. But the best part was because I was little, sometimes he'd let me sit on the armrest and put my hands on the steering wheel while he was driving back home to Virginia.

## Mom's Requirement #1: Self-Reliance

When my mother got her PhD in 1977, she worked at George Washington Hospital Center, setting up their transplant center. At the time, zero transplant centers existed in the United States.

Our mom was a career woman in the early 1970s, so her opportunities were not as broad as they'd be today. She was a powerhouse and let nothing stop her. It was around this time that our dad stopped being a presence in our lives.

Now, my mom reflects on our studiousness. "I'm a very serious person," she says, "and my son gets a lot from me. He has his way of doing things, and his way is a lot more interesting than mine. He makes sure he has time for himself, something he did even as a little boy. He always studied. I knew that—he always did what was required, and then some. I told them there's no excuse for not getting an A. You get these degrees, great, and you have to work the rest of your life. Just study and enjoy yourself."

In elementary school in Alexandria, Virginia, my mom got a call one day when I was in fourth grade and Resha was in third.

"The woman said, 'Do you mind discussing your children's future?'" she remembers. The teacher told her that Resha and I couldn't be with the rest of the class, and that we'd been tested, and we were going into ATP, the Academically Talented Program.

So Resha and I were in these accelerated classes with loads of extra work in fourth and fifth grade. The problem was, I might have been ADHD back then. I was bumping around and causing a lot of trouble. I was bored out of my mind! Back then there were no drugs for ADHD; instead, teachers increased your workload to keep you busy!

By then our mom had an enormously complicated schedule and a very serious life. She was executive director of the transplant center for the Washington area. She'd get a call at two in the morning and she would have to leave us by ourselves. She'd tell us, "Don't open the door to anybody."

We never did.

"They were both very mature," she says, adding that she had a beeper just for us.

## "The Resha" aka My Sister

Michelle aka Resha Jeneby is a year younger than me, and we both live for each other. I'm so proud that she's now an Assistant District Attorney in Woodbury, New Jersey. My sis is my heart; always has been. Even if I have a mischievous big brotherly way of showing it. That just keeps it fun.

"If he loves you, he will mess with you," Resha said during an interview for this book.

She remembers a love-hate moment from elementary school that remains forever seared in her memory banks. Here's how she remembers what happened:

"The ATP program had two classrooms, and we'd switch back and forth because we were in different grades. Well, one day we've got a sub, and when I go into the classroom he's just been in, I see my name on the board. I'm in third grade, so I feel a little panicked. *Why's my name on the board? Am I in trouble?* I wondered. Turns out, the sub had asked his class for the names of exotic or weird animals. Tayf (she calls me by my middle name) had said, 'The Resha,' so the sub wrote that on the board. I hit him when I saw him, and he thought it was the funniest thing. 'Why did you do that?' I said to him, and he just laughed: 'I called you a weird animal!'"

## Smart Kids, Smart Friends

"Honestly," Resha says, "our mother pushed us to be the top. She stressed studying and working hard, and our grades reflected it. Our friends were in ATP, and it was important to be with our friends, so we had to be smart like them."

Outside of studying, I was into Dungeons & Dragons, or D&D, a tabletop game that lets you play fantasy roles. I was also into computer programming with my Atari. *I was a straight-up nerd!*

Meanwhile, my sister was my constant companion.

"He treated me like a brother," Resha says. "He had to take me everywhere, even if he went skating. When he was in fourth grade, he became president of the school and I was vice president. That solidified people's knowledge that we were a team. Teachers liked it because we weren't bad kids."

We stayed out of trouble by focusing our brain power on computers.

Resha remembers, "We were writing code for computers and programs for DOS. We would write code to have the computer count from one to 10, skipping 2. We didn't have phones or TV like now, so we were always computer literate back then. We always played Atari together, constantly challenging each other."

### "Don't Lose Your Sister!"

Our friends knew we were a unit, which was a good thing because Mom's refrain was, "You're taking your sister."

Resha remembers that well. "Because I was only a year behind, I wasn't a stranger. So, we went to his friends' houses, and everyone responded to me with, 'Oh, okay.' I'd play Dungeons & Dragons with the younger brothers; there weren't so many little sisters. We'd be like a foursome. He was allowed to go places without me, but mostly he had to take me. He had to feed me. He had to walk me to school. He had to wait for me after school. We were latchkey kids. He was my dad, my brother, my uncle."

Meanwhile, my protective role for my sister dictated the location of playtime with my friends. If I wanted to go to a friend's house for a sleepover, Mom said, "No, we'll have the sleepover at our house and Resha will be there and you will sleep next to her. Suck it up, Buttercup!"

Mom always told me: "Resha is your responsibility. You have

to take care of her." At the same time, she told Resha: "You have to listen to your brother."

This extraordinary responsibility for my sister extended beyond our daily lives. Our mom traveled a lot for work, and she took us with her because she wanted to expose us to the world and different people. Our grandfather was living in England, so we visited him there. She also took us to Heidelberg, Frankfurt, Paris, Austria, and other European places for her transplant meetings. Times were simpler back then.

"Don't lose your sister!" Mom always instructed me.

"Why am I the target?" Resha remembers wondering. "'He wanders, too!' But we didn't have any sense that this was not the traditional way of traveling; this was all we knew!"

Mom would give us money for lunch and send us on our way. When she had business in Florida, at barely 9 and 10 years old, we got to go to Epcot Center. We rode the monorail to Disney, went on rides together, and made our way back to the hotel at the time Mom said. *By ourselves!*

Our mom remembers this well, saying: "They were so well-behaved and mature. I'd say, 'Here's the money, take what you want.' I didn't have to worry. He was focused and very aware of his surroundings."

## Always Doing Quirky Stuff

Resha and I had to entertain ourselves. There were no cell phones, and TV was way simpler. Once when we were playing outdoors, I found a couple of things in the trash from my dad's practice.

*What the hell?* I wondered. It kind of looked like candy, so I ate a few.

Resha went inside and ratted on me right away.

Turns out they were birth control pills!

I would do weird stuff like that all the time! Resha and I would get so mad at each other. She'd throw things at my face, like bricks and rocks, as if they were Frisbees!

Resha was clumsy, and a couple of choice instances have stuck with me.

She tells the story: "One time when he was lying down watching TV on a low TV stand with his arms back behind his pillow, I dumped a bowl of Cheerios on his head. He yelled, 'MOM!' like a little baby! Another time I dumped a bowl of spaghetti in the salad. I'm very clumsy. To this day, he still says, 'That's why you spilled a bowl of Cheerios on my head! That's why you spilled spaghetti in the salad!'"

It might sound obnoxious, but it was regular, brother-sister hijinks, and we had a blast as kids. I wouldn't trade it for anything. We still mess with each other and I call her every morning at 5:30 a.m. to check in.

## High School Rocked

I loved high school, and thought I was living the life. First, I had a lime green Camaro. As soon as I could, I spent $99 to have it painted lipstick red. Another cool thing was that I had my own "apartment" in the basement of our house, while my sister lived upstairs with my mom.

I had my own entrance, and I could do whatever I wanted, as long as I adhered to Mom's two edicts:

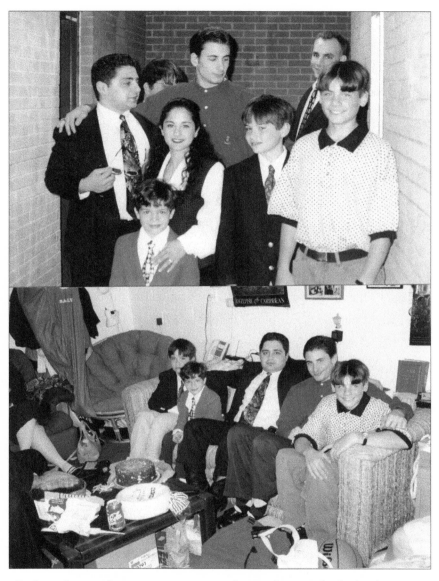

Resha and me with our cousins at my graduation from medical school in 1996.

1. Don't get in trouble with the police;
2. Get good grades.

My friends came over and partied, sometimes without me there! I was in great shape because I was on the wrestling team and I also pole vaulted.

My mom was so cool. She'd come down and check on everybody. She was very trusting and treated us like adults.

My lifelong buddy, Tad Fabian, and I met in high school chemistry class. Besides having a movie star name, Tad was an athlete—football, baseball, swimming—and my lab partner.

"It was probably a joke to him how easy it was," Tad recalls now during an interview for this book from his home on Marco Island, Florida, where he's a general contractor. "But he carried me through the class."

Tad remembers me being a low-key comedian, always having fun, but also knowing how to stay out of trouble. "He's funny, always this jovial guy. He has a wit. Quick wit and so easy to get along with."

Since we lived so close to DC, our school had a lot of nationalities represented. We just fit right in.

Tad remembers hanging out in the basement. "His mom didn't mind having people at the house—she'd be in and out. We went there after football games. Had a lot of fun. His mom trusted them to the utmost."

Tad remembers Resha being around all the time. "They were the picture of perfect kids: extremely smart and doing well in school at the same time. And they weren't getting in trouble or doing things they shouldn't be doing."

In high school, Resha and I hung in the same circles, the same crowd, the same friend groups. We spent a lot of time together.

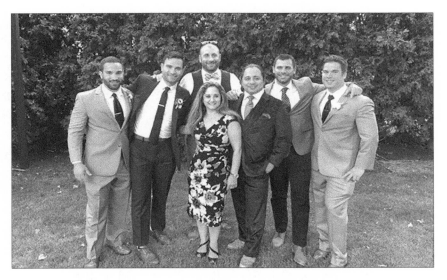

The cousins reunite (left to right): Sam Alarif, Nick Alarif, Chip Alarif, Resha, me, Matt Alarif, and Alex Alarif in 2017 at Nick's wedding.

Looking back, she says I really watched over her, starting in junior high. "He took me to parties, and always watched who I was with. He was very popular. It wasn't odd that we were always together. It was *Tayf and Resh*. We came from a whole family of doctors, and everybody knew the Jenebys were a very powerful family."

When I left for college, Resha's status instantly went up because she had a brother in college. Even though she had her own thing— she was class president and at the top her class—she'd come up to campus with friends, and that was always so cool.

She never did anything girly. Whatever I liked, she liked it, too. Her nickname was "Me, Too."

## Revenge is an Armani Suit

Remember the Toughskins we used to wear?

Well, when I returned for my 10-year high school reunion, I wanted to show everybody—especially those jerks who had teased me—that I had made it, and that I'd made it BIG!

So, I wore a tailored Armani suit. Custom suits were part of my life by then.

I was on a mission to find the girl from the political family who used to tease me and make me feel terrible. When I found her, she took one look at me, gasped, and exclaimed, "Holy, F! Is that you?"

I played it cool. "What's up? What's up?" I wanted to say: *Check me out, man! No more Toughskins!* But my suit said it all for me.

That was one of the coolest moments, ever! It truly exemplified the saying that, "Success is the best revenge!" It can push you to kick ass!


## Mom's Husband aka Dad

Our mom didn't date when we were in school because we were her main focus, along with her career. My father passed away when I was 11. My mom became Mom and Dad. And she was frightening!

"Once I came home," she recalls, "I was full-time there with them. I just wanted to make money to support them and care for them. I decided at the time that I would not get married again until they went to college. I didn't even go out. When they went out on weekends, I was involved. I even bought them cars. They gained responsibility, appreciated the things they had, and always paid attention to their grades."

When I was a sophomore and Resha a freshman, she met Thamir

AlHashimi, a widower with a son a few years older than me and a house in Hawaii. He was pretty smitten with her, but she wanted approval and permission from me and Resha.

"What would you think if I got married?" she asked us.

Resha was jumping up and down and excited for her. That was a yes!

I told her, "Mom, I'm very happy. Now I can sleep at night."

Thamir, when interviewed for this book, remembers, "A lot of people don't like their stepfather. But we just hit it off immediately. Interestingly enough, Tayf and Resha called me Dad whenever I was introduced to their friends, associates, and colleagues."

He says our mom did an amazing job raising us. "This is why I love their mother. Terrific kids. Never gave her any trouble. She had the determination, and she's no-nonsense. She said, 'Okay, I'll put you through college, I'll put you through medical and law school, but you have to perform. You don't get an A for effort.'"

Resha couldn't agree more: "She was never the typical mom. She didn't care what we were doing when we were younger. A lot of parents dote on their young kids when they're cute. Failure was not an option for us. She never got excited about anything we did unless it was academic. If Tayf was at the top in soccer, she'd say, 'That doesn't mean anything to me.' I was the top of the diving team in high school, and she'd say, 'So, what? You got into college? Got a job? So, what?' That's her way of saying there's more to your life. She'd ask of everything: 'What are you doing with it? Helping people? And are you happy?' She never had that with her mom."

Resha sums it up: "She ran us like a business. We had to produce. We got anything we wanted. Cars, a beautiful home, never had to worry about money, but we had to produce."

When Thamir came into our lives, he saw right away that Mom's main objective in life was to make sure that her kids succeeded and were well-rounded.

## A Huge Figure: Our Grandfather

My grandfather was a leader, a cabinet minister, a writer, a diplomat—a true renaissance man. He was gregarious, and he never worked under anyone.

My mom has seen her father's "open and out there" personality in me since I was a little kid. My grandfather had a super personality, always with an ego. She says I was a good-looking kid with golden hair. "Absolutely beautiful," she says with a loving tone that only mothers can make.

Her international trips gave us a chance to get close with our grandfather. I wanted to emulate him.

"I wish my father were here," Mom says. "He would have a ball with them."

She's right.

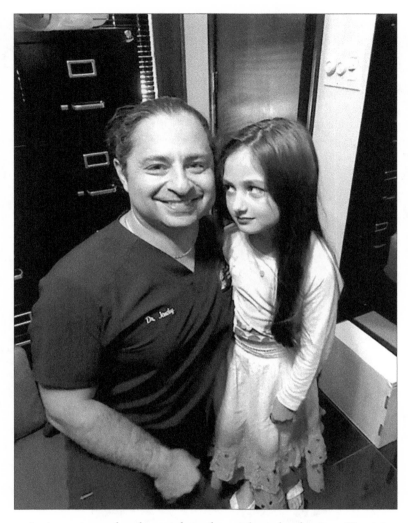

A picture is worth a thousand words—with my lovely niece, Kenzie!

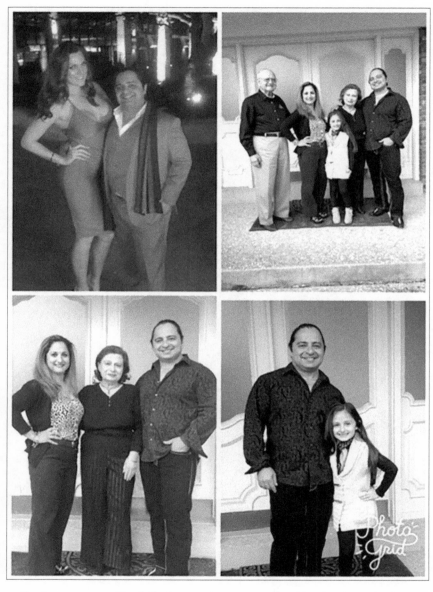

Smiles, everyone! Top left: Out on the town with Ashliegh. Top right: Dad, Resha, Kenzie, Mom, and me. Bottom right: Kenzie and me. Bottom left: Resha and me with our fabulous mother!

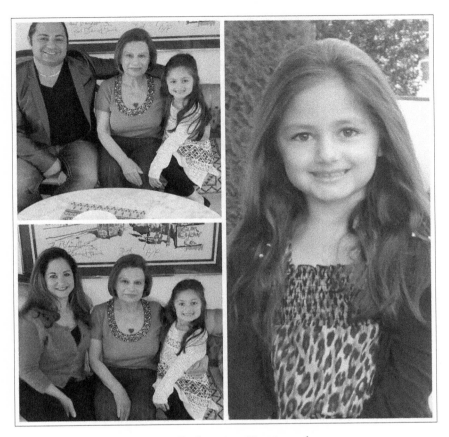

My mom, Resha, niece Kenzie, and me.

# 4

# College, Career, & Choosing Plastic Surgery

*"If life gives you lemons...*
*A simple operation can give you melons!"*

—*Anon*

W hat the hell is JMU?"

That's what my mom remembers saying when I told her I wanted to attend James Madison University in Harrisonburg, Virginia, about two hours from our hometown of Alexandria, Virginia.

"I thought he was going to go to Georgetown or George Washington," she says.

"It's just like Harvard," I told her. "All the smart kids go there."

I only applied to JMU, and got in.

"That's the kind of stuff he used to pull," Mom says.

She's right. Wait until you hear about the odds of getting into my plastic surgery program!

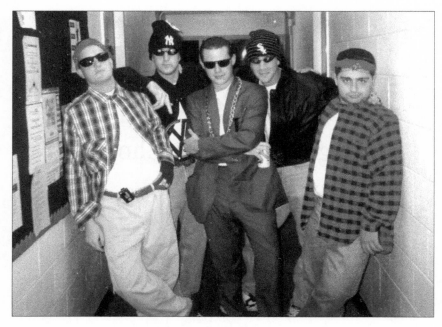

Wild'n'crazy college days!

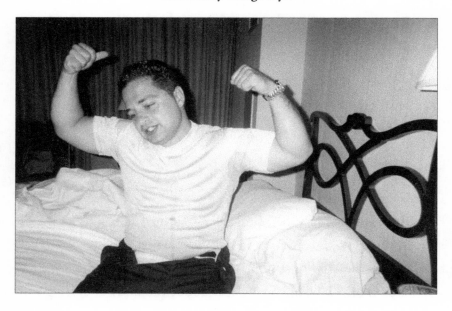

## No Room at the Dorm

Either JMU overbooked my incoming freshman class, or too many people said yes to admittance. In any case, the Office of Residence Life shuffled all the male students who needed to live in dorms, and I was part of the group of students who got to live at the Howard Johnson's Motor Lodge.

*I'm going to live in a hotel…? Awesome!*

I had two roommates, one studious kid who wore concert T-shirts and was on the "goth" side; and the other a neat-freak who used to fight with me because I'd always mess with him by moving his stuff. I was just being a jokester.

The general atmosphere at the HoJo was that of fun and mass consumption of alcohol. I wasn't a huge drinker, but after a while, I found myself with a beer in my hand a lot. Of course, we were all 18, so whoever stocked the beer would get 24- and 36-can cases. Somebody always had beer.

Soon everybody on campus knew, "Oh, you're the guys who live in the hotel."

Living in that hotel/beer-den/hang-out atmosphere made it hard to make good grades.

## Resha is *My* Sister

Resha joined me at JMU the next year. She was pre-med for her first two years, but she really sucked at organic chemistry. And she absolutely throws up when confronted by blood.

She was also a cheerleader, and one day someone said to me: "Are you Resha's brother? You're the cheerleader's brother?"

"Oh, no, no, no!" I told this idiot. "She's *my* sister!"

Then I tracked down Resha.

"He shut that down," she recalls. "'Uhuh! You're *my* sister.'"

## Volunteer Paramedic

I took an EMT class as a college course. I joined the Bridgewater Volunteer Paramedics, which was associated with the Bridgewater Fire Department in Bridgewater, a small town near the campus. The crew was made of paid guys from the town and some volunteers. I was good, so I got promoted to ambulance chief, which meant I could drive, sit, or watch.

The worst part of the job was the outfit: gray cargo pants and a white, button-down shirt. I looked like a dork! If I walked down Greek Row, where the campus fraternity houses were, I'd get sneers.

"Mr. Ambulance Man" and "Ambulance Boy" were the proper names when girls weren't saying, "You're the ambulance guy!"

Aside from the funny get-up, the experience introduced me first to what patients really are. Literally my first call was a motor vehicle accident along the highway.

We get on the scene, and it's a mess. Bodies everywhere, some cut in half. I'm seeing a tremendous amount of carnage *for the first time.*

I remember looking in the distance thinking I was seeing a stop sign. It turned out to be a person with his head buried in the dirt and with his feet up in the air. This guy had been thrown from his car and the force of his body hitting the ground had caused his head to dig a trench.

I didn't have much time to take it in—especially the bloating and lividity, or pooling of the blood in the upper chest and head—before someone yelled: "Jeneby, pull him out of the ground. Go dig him out."

*Oh my God,* I'm thinking. *This is my first contact with a patient ever—and it's a dead man.* I'd barely been in a hospital before this.

We loaded him into the ambulance and drove to the morgue. It was odd. I was thinking, *This is a little scary, but also kind of cool.*

For about a week after that, I couldn't get the smell out of my nostrils. It was a combination of rotting skin, feces (he had pooped himself), and the stench like the most foul-smelling meat you can imagine.

I volunteered every Wednesday from 1:00 p.m. until 7:00 p.m. After about six months, I was made crew chief. I remember thinking that the townspeople really took this seriously. This was their excitement. For me, initially, it was just a résumé stuffer.

The townspeople were local tradespeople, like a plumber or the guy who owned the hardware store.

This prompted ridicule that extended well beyond Greek Row; the townspeople used a condescending tone toward the smart college kids who were promoted quickly. They called me "College Boy" and it wasn't a compliment!

## Joining Kappa Sigma Didn't Exactly Help My Grades

People joined fraternities or sororities for an instant social life. One thing that kept bringing me back to fraternities was the fact that they attracted tons of girls. Pretty girls were everywhere!

My sophomore year, no longer living at the HoJo, I rushed a fraternity.

My first two semesters of college were a blast. I pledged Kappa

Sig, a meathead, athletic fraternity, and I was living in the frat house, partying my butt off.

My grades reflected how much fun I was having.

My GPA was 2.5.

I moved out of the frat house into a townhome with four other frat brothers, and then reality hit me.

*Oh, shit! I've got to get into medical school, and I've got a 2.5 GPA. I am totally under the gun!*

Oh, and those roommates? When we moved out, the place was trashed, and I learned a lesson.

"Why did you put the lease in your name?" my dad asked me.

How do I know NOT to put it in my name? Looking at the holes in the wall, I knew now!

## Ain't Too Proud to Beg—Once

*"Are you nuts?"*

That's what my mom said when she got wind of my grades.

"Tayf," she said, "What is this shit? If you don't straighten up, you're not going to get into med school. And I'm not going to support you."

She then reminded me that we are a family of education, on both her side and my dad's. My dad was one of 14 kids, 12 of whom were physicians.

My choices for med school were: first, the Medical College of Virginia; second, Eastern Virginia Medical School in Norfolk; followed by the University of Virginia, which was like the Ivy League of the South and at which I had zero chance of getting accepted.

I sat down with my mom and said, "How the F am I going to get into med school?"

Mom knew H.M. Lee, a transplant surgeon who was popular at the Medical College of Virginia, where 800 applicants were vying for 400 spots in the medical school.

She bought me a suit, and let H.M. know I was coming. I drove 130 miles to Richmond, Virginia, and met with Cynthia Heldberg, PhD, the admissions director at the time for the Medical College of Virginia and now Associate Dean of the medical school.

Basically, I got down on my knees, and said, "Please help me get into medical school. What do I need to do?"

I told her I'd been a knucklehead. I told her I had scrubs as a kid, that my toys were stethoscopes, and that everyone in my family was a doctor.

When I showed her my grades, she said, "It doesn't look good." Then she offered some reassurance by saying my only option was to get a 4.0 for the rest of my time at JMU. She also said I would have to get a really good score—a 30—on my Medical College Admission Test (MCAT), the computer-based, standardized test for prospective med students.

That sealed it. After that, I got serious: I had one 3.6 semester, and the rest were 4.0.

I even made the Dean's List in 1991 and the President's List in 1992. All four years at JMU, I was elected to Beta Beta Beta Biological Honor Society, which was a group of under-grad and graduate students who want to improve "the under-standing and appreciation of biological study and extending boundaries of human knowledge through scientific research."

When I took the MCAT, I got a 29. I was kind of a knucklehead. I got serious, but maybe I just didn't take that test well.[1]

I sent out 30 applications for med schools, and MCV was my first choice.

About two weeks after I sent the application, I got a letter saying they were going to look at my application.

*Relief!*

Three weeks later, I called to learn my status.

"We can't find your application," they told me.

*"Excuse me?!"*

After some digging, they told me, "Your application's been pulled."

"Pulled? What does that mean? It's been pulled and thrown in the trash?!"

"It's not here."

Come to find out that "pulled" in my case meant, unbeknownst to me, my mom's boss was an MCV alumnus and he called in a favor.

Getting into MCV was all my mom's doing. Without her, I wouldn't have made it into medical school. *She's made that painfully obvious for 22 years now.*

I was so excited. I flipped out. The whole family flipped out.

One thing I knew for sure: I was never going to feel like that again. I never wanted to play catch up—ever!

*My grades are never holding me back again. F this!*

I vowed right then and there: *I'm going to work a billion percent harder in med school.*

---

1   https://beinvolved.jmu.edu/organization/tribeta

## Making A's in Med School

Although I was making some friends in medical school, my goal was to make A's. I had learned that if you make Alpha Omega Alpha Medical Honor Society, also known as AOA, you can basically interview at Harvard, Yale, Stanford, UCLA, and so on. Making Junior AOA meant being in the top 10 percent of the class. That meant, I had a one-in-17 chance of being in the top of 170 people.

I had to take 36 classes in my first two years, with a test every three weeks on roughly 10,000 pages of material. *Like, WTF!*

I had to work, starting with anatomy, embryology, histology. I wanted to become a surgeon, so I had to get A's in those classes, especially anatomy, since the basis of surgery is anatomy.

In my first semester, I got all A's, which was very cool because each time I got an A, I received a letter saying, "Congratulations, you received an A in this course."

I loved getting those letters in the mail, so earning A's became addictive!

After my first semester, I qualified to get selected for AOA. I was number 16 out of 17. I earned the equivalent of 32 out of 36 A's. I knew I could have done that as an undergraduate, had I not partied so much and been a knucklehead.

Now, ambition kicked in strong, and my head was spinning with what specialty I would pursue. First, I wanted to be a neurosurgeon, also known as a "neuro." I did all kinds of research on traumatic brain injuries, and I published a few papers on it. Then I wanted to switch to cardiac. Then transplant. *Thank God I didn't pick any of those three!* Those specialties require rigorous, long hours in the hospital, which I am not inclined to do!

At that stage of medical school, I still didn't know a lot about the reality of each specialty. I was still almost a layman. Nobody really tells you how it is. I think it's a cruel joke. I learned this the hard way as a medical student one day during cardiac surgery rotation.

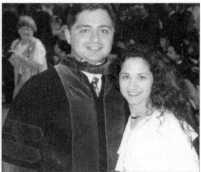

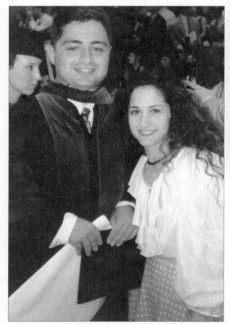

With my awesome sister, Resha, at my med school graduation— they make the doctors wear green for money.

## Can I Crack the Chest?

I was a lowly med student in the OR with the Chairman of Cardiac Surgery at MCV, his fellow, an intern, a resident, and the list went on. I was behind the fellow and the resident in the pecking order, so if anybody got to do anything during that surgery, I was fourth in line.

The procedure ended up being nine hours long. Couldn't piss.

Couldn't say you're thirsty or hungry. I just observed as attentively as I could, thinking, *I'm not going to say shit.*

Afterward, the chairman said, "You performed well today."

*Huh?*

I didn't do anything but stand there. I quickly learned his statement meant: *You weren't a pussy.*

Every morning, I'd get up at 4:00 a.m. to get there by 5:00 a.m. to help the interns write notes. I had to help the interns in order to establish myself as a hard-working med student. It's a real dog-and-pony show. I worked really hard for a month. I told myself: *Suck it up, Bitch! You want to become a surgeon!*

My presence was known to Dr. Alberto Guerrati, who did a lot of heart transplants. He knew I'd been working really hard. He brought me into the OR. He asked me, "Tom, what is wrong?"

I'd been doing everything these asshole interns and residents wanted me to do—all of their "scut work" as we used to call it.

I looked at Dr. Guerrati, and said, "It's my last day. Can I crack the chest?"

Some residents in their fifth or sixth year had never "cracked" the chest—that means taking the saw and splitting open the sternum, getting access to the heart. If you screw up the movement by an inch you could cut through the heart or lungs.

"What?" he said, clearly surprised at my request. He paused, winked at me, and then said, "Saw to Tom!"

*Oh, shit! Oh, shit! Oh, shit! Oh! Shit!*

The resident and the fellow gave me the stink eye, like, "I'm gonna kill you when we leave the OR." They spend years waiting for this privilege, but they didn't ask: I did!

I grabbed the saw. I placed one end under the xiphoid at the lower end of the sternum. Then I said, "Saw on," and I started to push. The saw got stuck pushing upwards and to the right (towards the heart!), so Dr. Guerrati helped finish it with me.

I'm exploding inside, thinking, *HOLY FUCK! I just got to crack a chest.*

Later that day, at 11:00 p.m., I'd been up since 4:00 a.m., and Dr. Guerrati asked me to get an x-ray during our final rounds of the day. I did because, again, I was proving I was a hard-working team player.

While I was gone, the story goes that Dr. Guerrati was talking to the resident and the fellow, when he said, "Jeneby's the hardest working med student. I let him crack the chest."

*"You did what?"*

They were still pissed. Air shot out of everyone's lungs.

In his Argentinian accent, he said, "I was a scared as shit, but I let him do it anyway."


## Dr. Isaac Wornom III

Dr. Isaac Wornom III is one of my heroes. I'm so honored that he wrote the Foreword for this book and agreed to an interview about what a great influence he's been on my career.

"I was a young faculty member in the MCV division of plastic surgery," he recalls. "We used to give oral examinations to students who were on their third-year surgical rotation. Tayf was assigned to me to give him his exam. He came in. I gave his oral exam. I thought he was very bright, and he did great on the test."

Dr. Wornom started asking me about what I was going to do.

"Neurosurgery," I told him.

"Have you ever heard of plastics?"

I hadn't. Back in those days before reality shows and Instagram, "plastics" didn't have the highly respected reputation like cardiac and neuro. Cardiac surgeons and neurosurgeons were like the fighter pilots or the star quarterbacks on the hospital team. Plus, they have important positions on boards.

Plastics, on the other hand, were viewed as lightweights, or worse, greedy snobs. Nobody paid them much attention. You only called them when you needed them.

So, when Dr. Wornom asked, "Why don't you come spend a month with me during your fourth-year rotation?" I had to give it some thought.

I went, and it was great. I got to know him—and some of the other Plastic Surgeons there.

Dr. Wornom, who has an excellent, dry sense of humor, thought I was bright-eyed, had an upbeat personality, and liked to talk to people. That's a big part of plastics—talking to people during consults—and relating to men and women from every walk of life.

What I liked about plastic surgery with Dr. Wornom was the diversity. One day we reconstructed an ear. Another day we did a breast augmentation. Then a cleft palate. And quite frankly, I'd read some books on Plastic Surgeons' income, and thought, *You know, if I'm going to support myself and the lifestyle I want, I could do it...*

## New Goals: USMLE & Matching

By this time, I didn't feel I needed to get more A's. I was now shooting for a high score on the US Medical License Exam 1. That's the test that medical students have to take to qualify for a license to practice medicine. It's required to get a residency; the higher your score, the greater your chances of getting matched with the most prestigious hospital of your choice.

The "match" process involves selecting your top residency programs (which have training hospitals) where you spend three to seven years working as a resident. The term "resident" comes from the old practice of requiring a doctor-in-training to live at the hospital. This essentially makes you a full-fledged doctor-in-training under the guidance of an Attending Physician. Residency is basically like a real-life class where you learn on live patients in a hospital.

So, in order to match for my top choice of a residency score, I aimed for a 90 percent or higher. I scored a 91! This score, along with my Junior AOA (top 10 percent of my class), meant I could write my ticket when seeking a hospital for my surgical residency. It was such a thrilling relief that my fate was finally back in my own hands.

A 91 on the MLE would get me considered by the top schools: Harvard, Yale, Princeton, Penn, Stanford, UCSF, and University of Texas Southwestern. When it was time to match, I was no longer a contender for neurosurgery. The neurosurgery match happened about three to six months earlier than the others, so I opted to pass.

I selected my top four schools:

#1 and #2: Harvard University and Brigham and Women's Hospital in general surgery;

#3: University of Pittsburgh for transplant; and

#4 University of Pennsylvania for plastics.

I went on 10 interviews thanks to my mom footing the bill for my flights, hotels, my suit, and spending money.

I had been to Harvard and Brigham, then I flew to Northern

California and interviewed at University of California at San Francisco. After that, I took a plane to southern California to interview at University of California at Los Angeles. Then I got on the last plane out, a red-eye from LA to Philadelphia, just in time for Philly's notorious 1995 snowstorm.

So, I'm on this red-eye and I stink. I haven't washed my suit. I've been living out of a suitcase, interviewing for two weeks, and now I'm sitting in front of a family with three, small, loud, crazy kids.

*No sleep, mofo.*

I knew I wasn't going to get any sleep before my interview. Here I am on my way to interview at a school that has one of the most competitive match odds in the system. Penn would only select two people: an in-house Penn person and an external, non-Penn person. I would be interviewing for the single external candidate's slot— along with 300 other applicants.

I was very fortunate that Dr. Wornom (a U Penn alumnus) had helped arrange an interview at Penn with Dr. Linton Whitaker, the Chairman of Plastic Surgery.

When the plane landed in Philly, I basically took a "whore bath" in the airport men's room. Wiped down with soap and throw-away towels so I didn't smell like a goat. Proceeded to my interview.

*I'm so tired!* I'm thinking, *Fuck it. Not a chance. I'm going against med students with Harvard and Johns Hopkins pedigrees.*

My hope dimmed even further when I saw my competition. One guy had co-invented some stent thing. These were some smart bitches! There I was, a public-school guy, trying to compete with these highfalutin Ivy League guys. They didn't know what to make of me. I felt like a mess, plus being sleepless, I was punchy, and cracking a few jokes. While they were super formal and taking this process very seriously, my lack of hope translated into a sort of a nothing-to-lose attitude that allowed me to be myself.

During the interview, Dr. David Low, a professor, made me draw my opposite thumb; he wanted to see if I was an artist. Sadly, my drawing was comical, like a stick figure. I did the best I could. Only later did I find out that he was actually a good artist—a runner-up—to become the drawer for *Netter's Anatomy* (the go-to book on anatomy). This guy would actually draw his notes—including arteries and veins—for the surgeries he performed.

Next, I went to Linton Whitaker's office. He was the Chairman of Plastic Surgery and a Texan.

"Dr. Jeneby, how are you doing?" he asked.

"I've been traversing the country to see you," I said, feeling foolish with fatigue. He had Scott Bartlett, the vice chair, and Donald Mackay, the craniofacial fellow, on either side of him. Bartlett was very obstinate, but Mackay was laughing at my jokes.

"Are you doing okay?" they asked.

"I'm doing okay, but this suit could probably interview on its own with the miles I've put on it," I said playfully.

*I couldn't believe I just said that.*

Scott Bartlett gave me a dirty look. Donald Mackay put his head down and chuckled.

I was sure that I had blown it.

Wrong!

When match day came, and all the schools announced their selections, I was shocked and thrilled.

I matched at Penn! I had finally made it to the big time!

*Oh, I'm going to be a Plastic Surgeon. Hahaha!*

Dr. Siebel was the head of the AOA at my medical school, and he was fond of me. "Sonny," he said with his Norwegian accent, "nice job. Ivy League."

"Penn's Ivy League?" I asked, shocked. This was news to me! I had no idea! I'm pretty sure I had mixed up Pittsburgh or Penn State with the University of Pennsylvania, when someone had said Penn Plastics.

Being oblivious to the fact that Penn is an Ivy League school, and only learning this on match day, made the news all the more amazing. In retrospect, getting accepted to Penn was the best thing I ever did.

## Don't Lose Your Sense of Humor

You have to understand that match day is a nationwide event for final-year med students. It's the day our fate is sealed for us. And given that I had chosen cardiac, transplant, and plastic surgery, my future really had been up in the air.

So, while the majority of people in my boat that day were feeling anxious, stressed-out, and concerned, my medical school friend and lifelong buddy, Brian Doyle, MD remembers that we chose to make it a light-hearted day.

"I wore a Mardi Gras T-shirt," recalls Brian during an interview from Tasmania, where he works for the Australasian College for Emergency Medicine. "Tayf wore a shirt that said, 'Some people think all I do is sit around and drink beer all day. Sometimes I throw up.'"

Brian says I had a lot of people fooled—or at least confused!

"He came across as this affable, kind of funny guy who didn't seem to take anything seriously," Brian recalls. "A lot of our fellow students were shocked to learn he was one of the best students. They were surprised he was in AOA."

Brian and I had been childhood acquaintances, and though he was a few years older, we hit it off when we were at MCV at the same time after he returned from some time off from traveling. He's been in Tasmania the last 15 years.

## I'm at Penn! Now What?

You buy a white coat. You get some scrubs from the hospital the night before. You're an MD. The white coat was the first time I saw Thomas T. Jeneby, MD.

I beamed!

6:00 a.m. report. The first instruction: *Don't fuck your shit up.*

We got a tour of the cafeteria, and we each got a beeper.

My first service was trauma ICU. These were some of the sickest people in the hospital, and I'm thinking, *I've never taken care of sick people.*

My beeper goes off at 7:01 a.m.

"What do I do?"

"Call that number," someone says.

A nurse answers, and blurts, "Dr. Jeneby, the potassium on so-and-so is 3.1."

I bust out this little book and look for potassium, then I take a shot in the dark: "Can you give her potassium?"

This nurse, and everyone in the hospital, knows it's the residents' first day. They want to teach us a lesson of who's boss.

I sense her sneering into the phone as she says, "How much, *doctor?*"

*OH, DAMN!* "What's normal?"

"Other people would say 20 milli repeat x1."

"Sounds good. Let's do that."

Sometimes they'd teach you things to sabotage you. Sometimes the attending would say, "Who the fuck ordered this? Jeneby!?"

I'd start to defend myself: "Well, the nurse—"

The attending wasn't having that answer. "The nurse!? You're the doctor!"

I was blessed to have a trauma fellow who was a general surgery grad take me under his wing. I guess he saw my animal tendencies, and taught me about drugs, labs, and how to set ventilators, so I could shine.

## Friends for Life: Anand C. Thakur, MD

When you're a first-year resident, your life is nuts. You work anywhere from 100 to 130 hours a week, sometimes not leaving the hospital for days. You really are a "resident," even if you have a mailing address across town.

One night while working late after a case was winding up, another resident and I had the good fortune of being in the right place at the right time.

Anand C. Thakur was an anesthesia resident at Penn.

"Our case was done," Anand said when interviewed for this book, "and the attending left; the residents left. We put on some dance music, and we both liked the song. We realized we were both off the next day. He was trying to go out; I was trying to go out. We were single and always on the lookout! Turns out, we were meeting different girls at the same bar. We met them together, and that started our friendship. We traded phone numbers, and instantaneously bonded. We'd go out, relax, have a few drinks, and be back at it at 6:00 a.m. When you work that many hours, you don't get to spend too many hours with too many people—so you value whom you spend it with. You don't want to spend time with people who irritate the hell out of you!

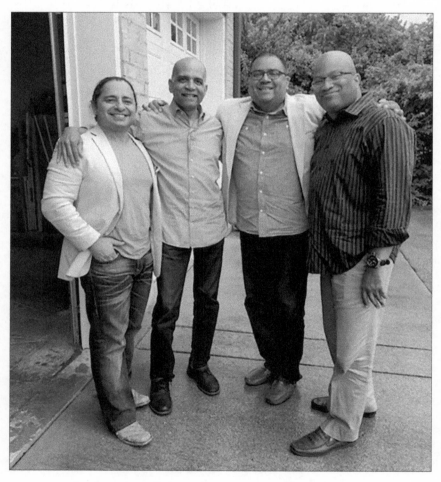

With my boyz (left to right): me, Dr. Herman Williams,
Dr. Anand Thakur, and Dr. Wayne Lee.

"That started our Friday night hang time, our guy time," Anand continues. "We'd go to a club, restaurant, and it was just guys being guys. We were a team. Saturday was girlfriend time. We would go out with them. We'd try to double date with them."

Even though he's from West Virginia, he's a Dallas Cowboys fan. That mutual interest, our insane schedules, and—loving football, golf, working out pretty heavy, and having a few drinks— made our friendship fun, strong, and enduring.

## Penn Offered Accelerated Program

When trauma ended, I went right into cardiac surgery. My first three years would be general surgery, then three years of plastic surgery. My program was exceptional; most regular programs were nine years. This highly-sought residency had you done in six!

Of course, the general surgery residents were kind of asses, and didn't really want to give me the time of day. They had a *Why bother? He's plastics*, attitude that made them not want to help me.

And I needed help. I was a terrible first-year resident, also called an intern. I didn't "round" very well. There's an overwhelming amount of data on 60 to 90 patients. I was being paid (about $2 an hour), but I was constantly sleep deprived since I was on call every third night. Sometimes I wouldn't leave the hospital for four days, even though I only lived a 10-minute walk away, on 24th and Locust Street in Philly.

## My First Surgery

I did my first surgery three months in. It was a breast biopsy with my attending and the senior resident.

*Oh joy, they are gonna kick my ass.*

The first several months, you don't get to do shit. You basically draw blood, get x-rays, and tend to the floor patients. "Scut work." It's the work that no one wants to do and because you're the lowest on the pole, you get these jobs.

I make the first cut around the areola. Even I know it sucked!

"God damn, Jeneby, are you plastics? What kind of Plastic Surgeon does that?"

*I'm only 26 and this is my first time cutting skin, damn you!*

I was shaking during the whole surgery and the attending and the chief resident yelled at me the entire time.

"Carve around this!"

"Stop the bleeding!"

"You suck real bad!"

"You sure you want to be a surgeon? Why don't you quit and go to family practice?"

*Kiss of death when a surgeon tells you this!*

I didn't know I could receive such a pounding for 40 minutes straight. When I tried to close the wound, I was shaking like a leaf. These two guys were humiliating the hell out of me, and it was tiring!

That kind of beating lasted 18 months! During my second year, someone underneath me got the beatings. By third year, I was in a surgery by myself for the first time—but it wasn't planned that way.

It was a colon resection for cancer. It was 7:30 a.m. and the patient was prepped. I had everything ready. We were all waiting for Dr. Morris, who was late. I beeped him.

"All right, Jeneby," he said from his Corvette, "open up. Pack the intestines. I'll be there in 20 minutes."

I'd never started a procedure by myself; I'd always had an attending there.

"Yes, sir," I said. I hung up the phone. My heart was pounding. I'd never made an incision by myself!

I turned around. Everyone was watching me, waiting for me to respond. It was like a slow-motion movie. And all I could hear was *Beeeep! Beeeep! Beeeep!*

The anesthesiologist pulled me back to reality when he barked: "What the fuck are you waiting for?"

Everyone looked at me.

*What the hell am I going to do?*

The nurse was having nothing of my moment either: "Let's get going. We've got a long day."

*This is nothing to them,* I thought. *I'm about to cut someone— holy crap!*

I moved in what felt like slow motion. I started the long incision at the top of her abdomen and then made a slow scalpel turn around her belly button.

When Dr. Morris finally walked in and saw my incision he roared: "You're a Plastic Surgeon?! What the fuck? Look what you did to her belly button!"

He yelled at me for about 20 minutes. During the whole procedure, he alternated yelling at me for 20 minutes then saying, "Good job."

## The Plastic Clinic

By the fourth year, I was doing plastic surgery only: six months with adults, six months pediatrics, and back and forth for my last three years. I saw a lot: a scalp torn off by an airplane; a motorcycle accident victim going 95 mph on the freeway who'd had half his skin scraped off; and a guy who'd shot himself in the face with a shotgun. The shot took off the front of his face by making his head tilt backwards but didn't kill him. It took 12 hours to put him back together.

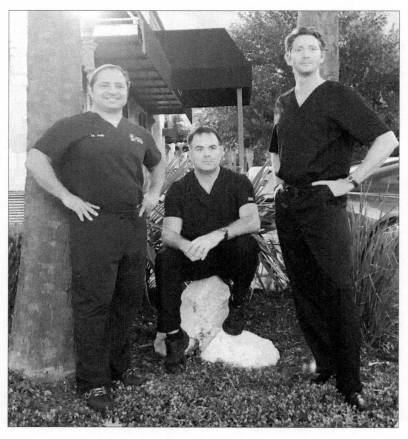

More of my homies: Dr. Eduardo Sanchez (center) and
Dr. Tito Norris on the set of a pilot series.

My last year, I was chief resident, and I got to work with the senior residents in the cosmetic clinic. This was a plastic surgery clinic that offered much lower rates than a board-certified Plastic Surgeon, because the surgeries were performed by senior residents. It was a learning clinic, but people would drive from Virginia, New York, Connecticut, and all over the East Coast to get work done.

I learned a lot at that clinic.


## No Fireworks; No Shooting Stars

On my last day, I just handed over my pager and walked out.

No bands, no fireworks, no shooting stars. No handshakes. No one said, "Thank you."

I just gave that place six years of my life, 130 hours a week, I was yelled at mercilessly, I got no sleep for days, and they're going to mail me a certificate...

And I just walked out...

I found a store and bought a new Nokia phone. Then I called my mom.

"I'm done. Now I've got to go look for a job."

In the meantime, I got some Chinese food from the food trucks outside of Penn, then walked to the nearest bar, where I had several Tanqueray and tonics (with a couple of limes). I called a girlfriend. She met me, went out, got hammered.

The next day, I got up and looked for a job.

# 5

# Arkansas?! Opening a Practice, Building a Brand

*"Annoy a Southerner and we will drain away*
*the moments of your life with our slow, detailed replies*
*until you are nothing but a husk of your former self*
*and that much closer to death."*

—*Maureen Johnson*

## Relocation: A Big Change

Al Capone. That was my dad's first thought when I said I was taking my newly minted, Ivy League-trained Plastic Surgeon self and moving to Hot Springs, Arkansas in 2002.

"We were a little surprised," my dad recollects now. "I knew Al Capone had run a gambling and prostitution ring in Hot Springs, and now they had made Tayf an offer he couldn't refuse. He'd traveled to Florida, California, Texas, North Carolina for interviews, but the fiscal conditions of the market were a little bit down. Job availability was not that great. But Hot Springs needed a Plastic Surgeon."

My mom remembers that I had offers, but I refused them, including one shady opportunity in Southern California.

"He had a good offer from some businessmen in Los Angeles," she says. "They were hiring Plastic Surgeons to do 30-minute breast augmentations or liposuction procedures. After he went to LA and met with them, he said, 'No way, Mom. I'm not going to work for these men who count surgery by the minute! That's not medicine. It's stupid! I've seen enough, and that's not me.' He also had offers from Boca Raton and some other places, but these offers would make him one of several people working for another doctor. He said if he was going to work, he was going to do it his way."

*I can't be someone's bitch.*

Frankly, the only person I wanted to work for was myself. Baptist Medical Center in Hot Springs offered to hire me to open my own practice. To get started, though, I'd benefit from the backing of a hospital system that would build up an office for me and give me a guaranteed salary the first year.

I had my mom's full confidence. "He was a young man," she says, "and he could adapt to anything. Even now, he will adapt to any condition."

I'm glad I had support because I knew I wasn't going to do it alone. My parents were retired, so I asked them to come with me to Hot Springs and help set up the business.

They jumped at the opportunity. They bought a condo in Hot Springs, but kept their home in Virginia, knowing the move wouldn't be permanent.

"They paid him a very handsome salary," my dad remembers, "guaranteed for one year. They built a clinic for him from a building that was there. Tayf gave them the model to build out of the shell, but he designed it. He wanted patients to flow through from one end to the other. I have to give him a tremendous grade for the way he designed it."

The coolest thing about my first practice was that at long last, I started using the same instruments I had been playing with at home, beginning when I was four years old. They were stainless steel, made in Germany, and they became my first operating equipment: suture holder, passers, scissors, retractors, and pickups.

## Day One in Arkansas

Along with setting up my practice, I was on call for two local hospitals for hand and face surgeries.

The craziness of those calls started on my first day in Arkansas. I walked into the ER in shorts and a T-shirt.

My cell phone rang. I stopped to answer it.

The woman on the line said, "This is Baptist ER. We're trying to call Dr. Jeneby."

"This is Dr. Jeneby," I said, thinking, *I'm standing in the ER and the ER is calling me…*

"We have a broken jaw for you to see," she said.

"Do I have privileges?" I asked.

Turns out I did have privileges, so I got to work on this guy who was a pimp with a broken jaw. That's right: my first call out of Penn was a pimp with a broken jaw!

Apparently, this pimp was in the ER after one of his prostitutes hit him on the side of his face with a baseball bat.

It'd been about three to four months since I'd worked on anyone, because of the time I took to take medical boards, move, and just get ready.

So, I got back in gear fast. First, I called the Stryker rep about getting a trauma facial set.

"I'm a new plastics," I told the rep. "I need you to come help me."

I ended up doing a great job on the pimp, including wiring his jaw shut for good measure. That may not have been absolutely required, but I felt it was necessary to keep this guy's jaw in place, and to give him a good two weeks to keep his mouth shut.

Did I mention that this was my first day in Hot Springs?

## Day Two in Hot Springs

The following night, I was further inducted into the reality of Hot Springs, with its picturesque lakes and round-the-clock outdoor activities.

Apparently, a big thing was playing on a water trampoline in the middle of the lake. At night. Under the influence of alcohol.

Fast forward: a guy is brought into the ER after having caught his nostril on a rusty nail protruding from the trampoline. He had an open nose fracture, and a messed-up forehead all the way into his hairline. He'd come down from about a 10-foot bounce.

I get to the ER at one in the morning, and I'm thinking, *You got me out of bed for this?!*

I put him back together in about six hours.

Afterward, I was feeling a little scared. My first two cases involved a pimp and a drunk guy doing stupid things in the dark in the middle of a lake.

What would my future hold for me in Hot Springs?!

Well, my next case seemed to follow the theme of this-is-what-I-signed-up-for.

An 18-year-old kid about two or three months into his career as a professional bull rider had gotten bucked off his bull. Once down in the mud, the bull kept stomping and his left rear hoof came down on this kid's face. The kid had come into the ER on a stretcher off the ambulance with the right side of his head facing down and his right eyeball on the stretcher. His eye socket was crushed.

*Nothing makes me more nervous than eyeballs out of their sockets!*

I called ophthalmology, reconstructed his eye socket, and got his eye back inside, though it was swollen completely shut. He was a bruised mess, but he was going to heal.

"When can I ride again?" he asked me.

"Bro!" I said, "you have a broken rib and tons of titanium in your face. You almost lost your eye. You can't ride again."

He looked straight at me, and said, "That ain't gonna work. What can I sign so I can ride again ASAP?"

*18-year-old kid. Gotta hand it to him.*

I told him he could sign an AMA, meaning "Against Medical Advice." He did. And he probably got back on that bull as soon as his eye opened—or maybe sooner.


## "We Were Just Messing Around!"

Even though I was on hand and face call, one beautiful day I was out enjoying some time riding around in my convertible BMW when I got a call.

"Hey, Jeneby," the ER doc said, "you need to come see this guy."

"What's going on?"

"He came in for diarrhea."

*Say what?* "Why are you calling me? Call the GI doc." I knew they often called me because I was highly trained, gregarious, and I could fix things.

"Just please come in," he said. "You won't believe it if I told you."

I walked in the room and saw a scruffy mountain man. One hand was normal. The other was huge, about three times normal size.

"What the F happened to your hand?" I asked, realizing it was hand-related after all.

Mountain Man shook his head. "I don't know, doc. I was bit by one of my rattlesnakes like four weeks ago."

"Oh, my God," I blurted in full stunned mode, not even catching myself to put on a poker face. "You have a pet rattlesnake?"

Meanwhile, I was looking at his hand thinking, *This doesn't resemble a hand.* His fingers were blown into these huge sausage digits. The skin was broken from the pressure of the swelling, weeping pus, and it was clearly infected.

The hand was in the process of dying because it was loaded with rattlesnake venom. I worked on him, but ultimately, he had to be helicoptered to a hand center.

During my calls, I saw a lot of people after boating accidents. Most often, alcohol was involved which, on the positive side, numbed the pain of a leg that's been cut on a propeller or whatnot. I saw people who'd been run over by a boat as a joke.

"What happened to your leg, dude?"

"Oh, my buddy... we were just messing around and he ran over me with his boat."

"We were just messing around," generally followed my standard question, "How did this happen?"

The upside to all these gruesome cases was that I had to save pictures to present my best six cases to my oral boards examiner. I had no shortage!

## Building A Practice

Human Resources in Hot Springs, frankly, were unlike the East Coast. Fortunately, I didn't have to deal with that since my mom was handling interviews, hiring, quality control, quality assurance, and designing an HR manual and employee handbook.

My dad called staffing a clinic with more than a dozen women "almost next to impossible. Women somehow, some way, seem to get combative."

Mom adds, "They get jealous of each other. We bit our tongues and handled them calmly."

Since I didn't have to handle the staffing directly, I could stay calm.

From my mom's perspective: "He doesn't get mad. He doesn't lose his temper. Yet he knows what's going on. I lose my temper, which is not nice. He had an even temper. Never heard him yell or scream. He's very understanding."

My dad organized the business. He's type A, OCD, and doesn't let a single detail pass him by. On the other hand, I'm a really happy-go-lucky type A personality. This caused some very tense and funny moments, but it was all for a good cause and in the spirit of family love.

"I ran my business," my dad says. "It was a multi-million-dollar corporation, and I had 176 people working for me. Tayf learned a lot from me. I'd tell him, 'This is how it is,' and sometimes he'd say, 'But, Dad, that was in your day. Things have changed.'"

This was the first I'd been with my parents in a long, long time. We were in a foreign environment and our task was huge.

As Mom puts it now: "He had a problem of building a name for himself. His competition was another doctor *born and raised* in Arkansas. In the end, he gave that guy a run for his money."

The three of us strategized at their condo every night over dinner.

How was I going to break through? We decided I would sponsor events in the office. We decided I would advertise in traditional ways—mailers, print, TV, radio—but also make my presence known everywhere I could. Any time there was an event in town, we would get a table, and pack it up with freebies. We did this at least two or three times a month.

We did so much that my outsider personae as the Yankee Doctor set me apart. People even said to my dad, "Oh, you're the father of the Yankee Doctor."

We worked awfully hard.

My dad remembers, "He did a lot of free consultations. He also did a lot of volunteer work with various organizations in Hot Springs. I remember there was a man who worked demolishing houses who had just gotten hit in the face with a wrecking ball. Tayf reconstructed his entire face and didn't charge a cent for it."

Mom adds, "He told the man, here is a bill to show you the work I did, but you are not obligated to pay. This is free."

This guy sent me $100 a month for 10 years, even after leaving Arkansas.

## The Yankee Doc

When I got to Hot Springs, I assessed the landscape. That is, I got the lowdown on the competition. Turns out, Baptist had been using a team—a young guy who was a native Arkansan, meaning he lived, breathed, and ate Arkansas—and an older Plastic Surgeon who had recently been taken out of commission. The reason? He could no longer perform surgery because a nerve in his hand was nicked while he was getting a carpal tunnel release. The older guy sold his practice to the younger guy.

So, it was that guy and me, the Yankee.

He had a giant head start and the benefit of assuming the role as the dude in the practice. He was a local. He was a known commodity in the community.

I looked at what he was doing, and I came up with my own ideas.

My mom says of my marketing skills, "He's uber-creative."

And my dad says I'm still creative to this day.

Marketing is fun for me. The object is to win, and I love winning. When I wasn't working, I was studying marketing.


## Good Times

Coming from Philly, where there was a bar on every corner, finding fun stuff to do in Hot Springs as a single doctor left a lot to be desired. I quickly discovered that folks would come down from the surrounding mountains on Saturday night and hang out at Wal-Mart. *I'm from the East Coast, WTF.*

I lived in a condo on a lake and had my own dock. I bought a boat and made my own fun. After all, Hot Springs was beautiful.

One of my buddies from those days is Eric Guilliams, who's now a urologist in Springfield, Missouri. He doesn't remember the specifics of our meeting, "but I do remember that day. I came home from the hospital and told my wife, 'I met someone today, and we are gonna be long-term, good friends.' I grew up in the South, but went to college with a lot of Northerners, and have always been intrigued by their blunt/straightforward/no bullshit approach to things. Thus, my close friendship with Tayf. This Yankee was a total fish out of water in Arkansas. That being said, don't let his over-the-top, aggressive personality fool you: underneath that is a guy who would do anything for a friend."

Eric remembers going duck hunting with me. "Imagine *him* with a shotgun, cammo, and waders," he says. "I can't remember what he was saying, but I remember laughing the whole morning."

We were colleagues, so we got to see each other at work, too.

"One time I walked into his OR and said 'WTF' way before WTF was a thing," Eric says. "For some bizarre plastic surgery reason, he had just surgically connected some woman's arm to her belly. I remember saying, 'Are you f'ing kidding me?' His response? 'What, bro?! It's a real procedure—I swear!'"

It is!

I was only around 32 years old in Arkansas, but Eric remembers that I used to joke about someday having a young, hot wife. "Tayf would always say, 'I went by the hospital nursery today to check on my future bride.' Still cracks me up."

Eric remembers, "He had an awesome BMW M3 convertible. I loved it so much, I eventually bought one myself! One time it was in the shop. Much to his dismay, the only loaner available was an old, ugly Toyota Corolla. With the greatest respect to all the Toyota owners out there, I still laugh when I think about when he came to our house in his trademark Italian suit, long hair, and shades, and said, 'Yo, check out my high-rolla Corolla!'"

Eric adds, "I am proud to say I am in a small group of people who understand this larger-than-life, crazy man, and I miss him."

Eric and I formed a company to buy a bar on one of the lakes that had ridiculously good boat traffic. But before we did anything, the place got raided for drugs, and was shut down. That would have put a terrible spin on my whole Arkansas experience—and my parents would have killed me!

## Doing Laser Hair Removal—and Not Doing Laser Hair Removal

I bought a laser hair removal machine as a way to enhance the business. Since I was the surgeon, I was using the machine myself on patients because I didn't really have the staff to use it. I was doing bikinis, underarms, and so on.

Well, the head of staff at the hospital, a cardiac surgeon, befriended me. He was a super-likable guy, and in the small town of Hot Springs, pretty much everybody trusted him.

This guy and I went out to dinner a few weeks after I'd done his wife's bikini line.

Our dinner started fine. He was drinking a lot, then our dinner came, and two hours into a rollicking good time, he got serious, and out of the blue he asked, "Did you like looking at my wife's *pussy?*"

*Woah, woah, woah!*

I'm floored! This is more than a little odd.

"Holy shit, man," I said. "Hold up, bro. I didn't know you were like this about that. I'm a doctor like you, remember?"

The next day, I trained my medical assistant to do hair removal, and I never touched a hair removal machine again. *Lesson learned.*

## I'm Not Going to Die in Arkansas

After putting in 16 hours a day for around eight months, it became clear to me that Hot Springs, with its carnage, weird behaviors, and lack of personal safety initiatives, was not big enough for my dreams. Ultimately, I was going to move to a bigger, more cosmopolitan city.

When I moved to Hot Springs, I knew I would not die in Arkansas, but I didn't know how quickly it would take to get to that point.

In a relatively short period of time, I'd captured almost 40 percent of the market in Hot Springs, and I knew I literally had no place to go if I stayed. I had to find a bigger city.

The point of expansion for the business was limited because Little Rock, only an hour away, had a huge number of Plastic Surgeons. My competition locally may have been one Plastic Surgeon, but we were both competing with University of Arkansas physicians. People all over the state went to Little Rock first.

I remember sitting with my mom and dad on multiple occasions, strategizing how to grow bigger and bigger, and realizing as great as my marketing was going, I was not going to go further than I'd gone.

It was time to go.

## San Antonio Calls

Baptist in San Antonio, by chance, was offering again: a salary for one year, build up a practice, and pay them back. Same deal, only in a market which my mom recalls, "sounded a lot more attractive than Hot Springs."

# 6

# Success Secrets of a Marketing Machine

*"Failure is the key to success, each mistake
teaches us something."*

—*Morihei Ueshiba*

I am a marketing monster.

You might look at me—an eccentric guy with long hair who works on boobs and butts all day—and think I'm not as business savvy as an MBA.

Wrong.

I'm a numbers nut, an analytics junkie, and a fiend for the latest information about marketing, especially new social media platforms, and how I can use them to promote my business.

*I learned this the hard way.*

Marketing has been an obsession of mine since I opened my business in Arkansas. Staying on top of the hottest trends—along with having the balls to be super innovative—has enabled me to attract a ton of new clients, as well as boost my bottom line year after year.

"Dr. Jeneby is a marketing genius," says Ana, my full-time marketing assistant. "He reads the Harvard Business Review, and gives us books, articles, video news reports, and everything that has to do with social media, print marketing, different apps that are coming out, and the latest information that can help us improve our marketing. He's a sponge and wants to read and know everything."

The last Friday of every month, Ana and others on my staff of 21 are required to do a book report on an article or book pertaining to the type of work they do in the office.

Ana has to read, study, and write about new information that can help us improve how we promote our products and services.

"Knowledge is power in this office," Ana says. "Education is key here. He encourages me to learn from other people—and learn a lot!"

## Data + Analytics = Improving our Performance

I do 14 surgeries every week. Each time I take one of these patients into surgery, I complete a hand-written form that asks for:

- Patient name

- Procedure

- Referral source

- Amount collected

Before the patient gets prepped for the procedure, I ask him or her, "How did you hear about us?" Usually it's a multitude of different sources. I'm usually amazed at the number of different places people hear about the practice.

Then I want to know how much money we're making on the procedure.

That's how obsessed I am with analyzing all our data to determine which promotional platforms and referral sources are drawing in what types of procedures, and which are the most profitable.

Then I can say, "We got three patients from Facebook: one got boobs, one got a tummy tuck, one got a blepharoplasty. We got two from KISS Radio: one got boobs, another got lipo."

My motto is, "Show me the numbers!"

My marketer collates the data and presents it in a PowerPoint presentation during our marketing meetings every Tuesday morning before we open to see patients.

"Dr. Jeneby is a big numbers person," Ana says. "If they don't add up, we try something else. If it's not working in one area, he's eager to change things."

We work hard at marketing, so we can make our Center look like a fun, friendly place to get the safest, most advanced procedures. Our live social media broadcasts have revolutionized our marketing strategies, because they literally give people an inside look at the mysterious, fascinating, and sometimes scary world of plastic surgery. They see everyday people getting successful surgeries in a great environment.

When people watch our broadcasts on live social media, we're playing cool music in my private operating room, and we've got Ana broadcasting live on Snapchat with hearts floating across the screen, and another staff person has us live on Facebook. At the same time, I'm describing the procedure and answering our viewers' questions, while paying strict attention to the austere safety measures that I take to prevent infection and errors. All while my anesthesiologist constantly monitors the patient's vitals. Safety is the key to success; the fact that we make it entertaining attracts national media attention.

*Inside Edition* has done many feature stories about me. One story in particular on the popular TV show was called, "Meet the Cosmetic Surgeon Who Livestreams His Procedures for All to See: 'It's Show Time.'" It aired on September 6, 2016 and showed how I perform surgeries live on social media. *Inside Edition* cameras were in my OR as I performed a breast aug on a 32-year-old mother and wife, and my staff was broadcasting live on Snapchat and Facebook.

Like all patients who appear on live broadcasts, the woman gave us permission in advance. Some patients actually request that their procedures be broadcast. That way, their friends, family, and all the world can watch, and have fun seeing the "before" and "after" pictures, which I often post on Instagram.

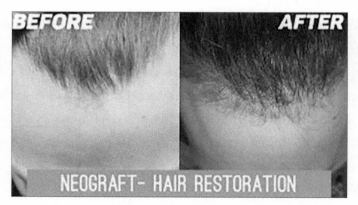

**Billy Hair Don't Care!**

For me, being featured on a national TV show three times is a promotional dream! It casts me as an expert in my field, showcases what I'm doing that's unique, and creates a celebrity aura that hooks people in.

Without a doubt, our aggressive and innovative approach to marketing is a major factor to running my successful plastic surgery center and spa.

In addition to having my dedicated, in-house marketing assistant who answers to me and deals with 10 outlets of marketing, we also employ a local PR firm (Sammis and Ochoa) and a national public relations firm that orchestrates the Search Engine Optimization (SEO) and blogging to boost the rankings and visibility of our website.

I also hired videographers to make video stories for YouTube featuring my patients' journeys, starting from pre-surgery, through the procedure, then six weeks to three months after.

Marketing has become a lot more advanced for me in recent years. Here's a peek at some of the other things we do.

## Dr. Jeneby on Radio and TV

Television is one of the many marketing tools and tactics that we use every day. I used to do much more traditional TV marketing, and back in 2007, I was one of the few Plastic Surgeons who used TV marketing. Before that, I started out just marketing in newspapers and the Yellow Pages. The advent of social media has revolutionized our promotions, especially over the past two years. More on that later.

For now, TV is still an important element in our marketing strategy.

In business and in life, relationships mean everything. You have to build good relationships with people in your personal and professional realm, because that forms a foundation of trust and camaraderie that translates into win-win situations for everyone involved.

This is very true in the media world. It's come really naturally for me to meet key people in radio and television, and it's been almost organic how we've created friendships and associations.

This couldn't be truer than my personal and professional relationship with bad-ass radio show host Billy Madison. He is San Antonio's answer to Howard Stern, and his top-ranked, nationally syndicated morning show reaches 500,000 people in San Antonio daily and countless others (in syndication) in California, Maryland, Washington, Florida, Oklahoma, and Texas, as well as having 136,151 followers on Twitter.

My weekly "Ask Dr. Jeneby Anything" spot on the Billy Madison Show brings some titillating content to his program, as listeners call in to ask about boob jobs, butt lifts, lipo, man boobs, lip-plumping fillers, Botox, you name it. I get to promote my business, while he gets to entertain and educate the men and women who tune in. Plus, his two co-hosts, Derek and Nard, have a field day indulging raunchy dude talk in reference to breasts, booties, vaginal rejuvenation, and, well, you can just imagine the scurrilous territory where some of these conversations end up. It's hilarious!

I'm known as "the Plastic Surgeon to the Billy Madison Show," or "Hands of God" as they jokingly refer to me, which airs on KISS 99.5 FM in San Antonio.

Listeners call in with questions about everything I do, and I share the latest specials that we're running. In October, for example, I sat in the studio with Billy and his crew and talked about our "Booo-Beee" Halloween special.

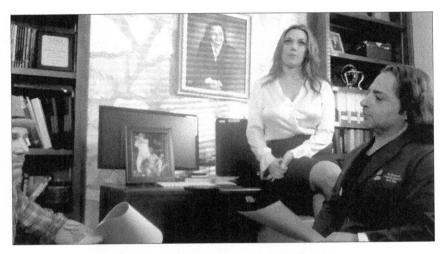

**Kickin' it with Ashliegh and Billy Madison at a TV pilot.**

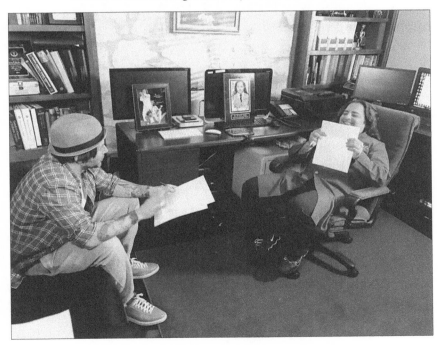

My relationship with Billy and his crew has become so great, they and their wives have come to me for procedures, which I've broadcast live on social media. First, Nard brought his wife in for new boobs, and we posted snippets of the consultation and procedure on our social media platforms. Second, Billy has come in for our cutting edge, NeoGraft hair implant procedure, and it's all documented on my Facebook page. He also gets Botox, Laser Resurfacing of his face, and fillers.

A video I posted on February 16, 2018, using my new "Dr. Jeneby Presents" logo showcases Billy's NeoGraft journey at Spa Black.

It starts with me in a suit, my hair down, and I'm talking about how I asked the NeoGraft company for permission to make Billy Madison the spokesperson for the product because he's syndicated on the radio and he's in the perfect target demographic that the company wants to reach.

Voilà! That got Billy talking about it on the radio, saying, "I'm trying to become the spokesperson, the champion if you will, the one who rides in on a horse and tells everyone about it."

He also agreed to let us film his entire procedure.

"Doc offers financing, so like, dudes will spend six grand on their wives' breasts, but they'll forget about themselves," he says, wearing a surgical cap with a purple line over his forehead where we are about to implant hair to restore his hairline. "Make men hot again!"

He is on Valium and is really talkin'!

He also talks about how it's painless and life-changing as we harvest hair from the back of his head and implant it in front to restore his receding hairline.

Throughout the 4.5-hour procedure, he's talking about how good it feels to be lit on the pain-killing medication, and he's rambling on about "my friend Oprah Winfrey."

"Are you really friends with Oprah Winfrey?" I ask.

"No," he admits.

We are all laughing. Then he tells us about his friend's mom who was not wearing a bra while she gave him a haircut.

After the procedure, we film Billy holding three boxes of products to take home.

"If you're losing hair, Dr. Jeneby will be there," he says.

I explain that we spent nearly six hours together, using 1,000 grafts in his anterior hairline to fill in the temporal areas. Then I ask him how he feels about it.

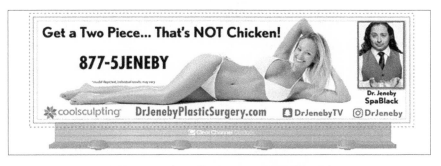

You're looking at 672 square feet of pure sexy on a billboard in San Antonio!

"I've had the most phenomenal week," Billy says as I'm sitting beside him in my scrubs. "Not only did I get my iPhone 10, but now I've got, like, hair! Thanks to this guy. This guy honestly is one of the kindest, gentlest, most handsome-haired men ever. I mean, it's gonna be fantastic."

He went on to say, "It's gonna be awesome. NeoGraft hookin' me up with hair. Thanks to this guy, Dr. Jeneby, Hands of God. If you're a dude out there, and you're losing your hair, you don't have to. Don't be ashamed. I'm proof. Talk to this guy. He's got financing available. NeoGraft. Get your hair back. Did I mention he offers financing?"

This kind of marketing is powerful for a lot of reasons. First, the patient is a celebrity, so people watch because they love Billy. He's funny, and they want to follow what he's doing. It's also pretty cool that he has the *cojones* to undergo a cosmetic procedure on live social media.

Second, the videos explain to viewers exactly what the procedure involves, so this demystifies it and eases people's fear about whether it hurts or whether it's effective. At the same time, Billy Madison's personal experience and endorsement of the procedure are worth their weight in gold. People admire him and trust him. The message becomes, "If Billy Madison is confident enough to allow Dr. Jeneby to perform this procedure on him, and he's praising the process and the results, then I can trust Dr. Jeneby to bring me good results, too."

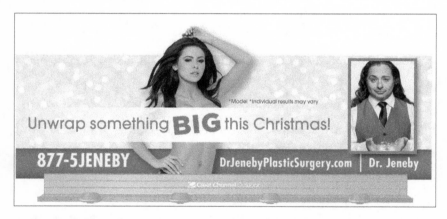

**Another billboard. No one ever accused me of not having a sense of humor!**

The experience gets even more play when Billy goes on the air to talk about the procedure that I successfully performed on him that's now making him look and feel better and younger.

Whether it's live video of Billy Madison getting hair implants or a woman undergoing a breast enlargement or Brazilian Butt Lift or a dude having his man boobs removed, the viewers on social media are getting educated on what exactly each procedure involves.

This is the educational component of the social media phenomenon. It was never our intention; we started using Facebook, Instagram, and Snapchat strictly as promotional tools. But these platforms have evolved into "educational marketing."

People can watch and say, "Oh, that's a tummy tuck? That's not so bad. You make it look easy."

The OR is a mystical place. People have heard about it. They've seen it. They don't know too much, and it's real scary. It's like the cockpit of an airliner. You kinda want to know what these guys are doing on takeoff, midair, and landing.

I make it more educational, less "spooky," and almost entertaining. People say, "I was watching. I wanted to do it. I was really scared, and then I saw your videos. Now I'm just not scared anymore."

I had no idea that social media marketing would have the side effect of easing fears. Of course, it pushes some people away, but overall, I think the effect is positive.

## "Dr. Jeneby Dancing with the Stars!"

What's another way I've leveraged TV appearances as a marketing tool to build a celebrity aura and name recognition? I competed in the televised *Dancing with the Stars San Antonio*.

Wearing an all-white outfit trimmed in silver rhinestones, I start solo doing a John Travolta-esque rendition of *Saturday Night*

*Fever*. I dramatically free my hair from my ponytail, and am joined by my scantily clad, professional dancing partner.

To maximize the impact, I hosted Dr. Jeneby's Dancing with the Stars event, with proceeds going to the show's beneficiary, a charity called Family Endeavors.

The event included a meet and greet with the crew from 99.5 KISS FM's Billy Madison Show: Billy, Derek, and Nard! We had live music and an appearance by The FABOOBLICIOUS GIRLS! Food, drinks, giveaways, raffle prizes, and event-only specials from the Plastic and Cosmetic Center and Spa Black. We also offered a chance to win a $1,500 gift certificate toward a regular-priced service at Spa Black.

We promoted the event on Facebook, and it was a blast for everyone.

My performance on *Dancing with the Stars San Antonio* was super fun and high energy. I even lifted my partner—Holly of the Arthur Murray Dance Studio in San Antonio—onto my shoulder!

My appearance on the show boosted my name recognition around town. A lot of people still think I performed on the national program and stop me on the street to chat about it. Participating in events like this has nothing to do with plastic surgery, but are mega-promotional opportunities, which of course we blew up on our social media platforms.

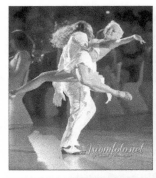

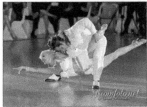

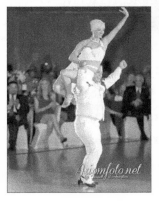

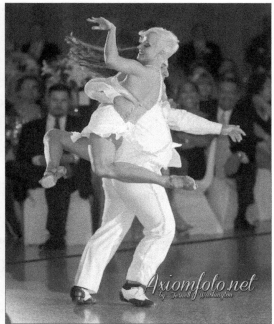

**Dancing with the Stars with my phenomenal partner, Hollie Simkatis. Photo credit: Axiomfoto.net by Terrell Washington**

## Social Media

Our overall strategy with social media is to stay uber-current. That means watching what's trending, offering specials that correspond with the seasons and annual events, and studying the latest and greatest in social media apps.

We typically post three to four times every week. Less is more; we don't want to bombard people, and we value quality over quantity.

We're finding that people love videos more than still photos, and they eat up anything I post about my personal life. Pictures and videos of me and my wife Ashliegh in cool places like Las Vegas, Miami, and New York get tons of likes and comments.

"People really want to see a day in the life of Dr. Jeneby," Ana says.

As for hashtags, we try to use different ones.

"We try to hashtag our products," my marketing assistant adds. "We also look at what's really trending or San Antonio. We go to Instagram and Twitter to see what's trending and go along with that trend. People will look at a hashtag one week and think it's interesting, and by the next week, no one is using it anymore. It's forever changing. We try different things all the time. With social media, there's something new or omitted almost every week. It's always evolving."

Likewise, my marketing tactics have been evolving considerably since I first started marketing my business in Arkansas. Since the middle of 2016, social media has dramatically changed the way we market the Plastic and Cosmetic Center of South Texas and Spa Black.

## Facebook

I started my Facebook page for Thomas T. Jeneby, MD, Plastic and Cosmetic Center of South Texas around 2007, and now have more than 60,000 fans; some of my Facebook posts reach a million people.

"I'm addicted to your Facebook Live videos," people tell me at parties. "I can't stop watching! It's fascinating."

Two of my favorite posts were the TV commercials we produced for Super Bowl Sunday in 2017 and 2018. During the days leading up to the big event, we really promoted the hell out of it.

"It. Is. Coming!" we posted. "In T-minus 24 hours, get ready for something big as you're watching the lead-up to the Big Game! Don't miss it on Sunday—get your TVs on by 4:15 p.m. to catch us on News 4 San Antonio!!"

With the post was a GIF from our Super Bowl commercial featuring my wife Ashliegh on one side of me, and my Spa Black technician Andee on the other, both kissing my cheeks at the same time, as they kick up a heel.

The next day, on February 4th at 5:31 p.m., we posted still shots from the super-sexy commercial featuring Ashliegh and Andee, both dressed as referees with lots of cleavage. I'm standing between them, wearing a black suit, and a white dress shirt with an open collar.

The post said, "🏈 Here it comes! Keep an eye out for my #Superbowl commercial for an AMAZING deal you don't want to miss!" along with #teamjeneby.

The commercial finally aired on Super Bowl Sunday. Then we posted it at 8:38 p.m., saying: "In case you missed it, here is my Super Bowl commercial with an amazing, limited time only, Mommy Makeover special!"

I love this commercial! It shows Ashliegh and Andee in their super-sexy referee outfits, both blowing red whistles.

"Personal foul, bikini zone infraction," they say in unison.

The narrator adds, "Summer bodies are made in the winter."

Then I stand between them and say, "So take the Jeneby challenge today and score right now with our beautiful game special. For a limited time only, a Mommy Makeover, which is a tummy tuck and breast augmentation, is only $9,999. Just text HOT to 38470."

The commercial continues: "So don't be penalized. Visit DrJenebyPlasticSurgery.com."

I wrap it up by saying, "And the next time you step on the scale…" then playfully remove my glasses and add: "…it'll say one hundred and sexy!"

BAM!

And on February 1st at 9:03 a.m., we posted a "before" and "after" picture of a 28-year-old "victim of family violence who was kicked, causing her IUD to tear into her uterus, requiring emergency surgery. She now has a terrible midline scar. We are performing lipo and scar revision to even out her abdomen. Please share to bring awareness! Thank you! Dr. J. and Staff!"

We included the hashtags: #probono #familyviolence #giveback #drjeneby and #drjenebytv.

After a Facebook Live broadcast of a breast aug on February 5th, we posted the 30-minute video at 10:31 a.m. The post said: "Adjustable Breast Implants!" and I describe the patient as 5'2" and 137 pounds.

On camera during the procedure, I say, "One breast is very asymmetric compared to the other one, so we're going to do different sizes on her implants, plus she gets an adjustable."

I explain how I'm developing the plane under the muscle to insert the implant.

*People are going nuts.*

"Again, if you have any questions, text 'BOOBS to 38470," I tell viewers.

Then I tell my surgical tech Britany that, "I was dreaming last night about when I was a resident at Penn. It was a little bit of a nightmare. I always have these dreams where I'm going back to school and studying again. You know what that is? It's like feelings of inadequacy. Doctors always have a small bit of doubt to make sure their dreams will go well. I have dreams of teeth falling out sometimes. It's a common dream. At 3:00 a.m., I wake up, looking up dream interpretations right then."

A close-up video shot shows the boobs with squares over the nipples. With the post we included:

32A->34D

Outpatient

18883jeneby

5999$ 45 Min Back to work 1-4 weeks

Snapchat: DrJenebyTV

Go see more videos on my YouTube: subscribe to: drjenebyplasticsurgery *individual results may vary * posted with patient full permission **We do not own the rights to any music in the video**

Text "BOOBS" to 38470.

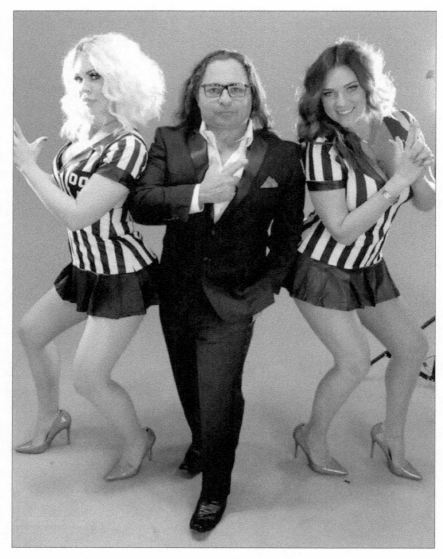

Super Bowl ad with Andee (left) and Ashliegh. The commercial ends by me wrapping it up: "And the next time you step on the scale…" then playfully removing my glasses and adding: "…it'll say one hundred and sexy!"

## Facebook + Snapchat = $$$$

We use Facebook, Instagram, Twitter, LinkedIn, and Snapchat all together, and they generate a lot of revenue for me. They're unique social media platforms that reach different demographics, who usually want distinct products and services. Most of our clientele is between 25 to maybe 50 years old.

On Snapchat, our target audience is millennials, who are 18- to 30-year-olds. Younger women want lipo and breast implants.

Our Facebook demographic is slightly older: the 35-and-up age group. Most older women are mainly seeking tummy tuck surgeries, Mommy Makeovers, facelifts, and higher-cost procedures. A typical patient who's 35- to 45-years-old has kids, and she wants our signature Mommy Makeover.

## Snapchat

When we film live surgeries, we have two smartphones in the OR. One is for Facebook Live, where we write a post, click "start my video" and we can stream for as many hours as we desire. Facebook is our top platform, where we have 60,000 followers. At the same time, we have another smartphone broadcasting on Snapchat, where you can find me as Drjenebytv. We also use Twitter and Instagram, which reach over 10-20,000 people!

Snapchat works great because it's short, 10-second clips where we can film a snapshot of the surgery, then add animations, different filters, and a little bitmoji that looks like me. With all these features, Snapchat is more entertaining. We can do a boomerang or cool little effects to add to our videos to make them more entertaining than Facebook, which is just video without any enhancements.

We also use Snapchat to show people a day in the life of Dr. Jeneby.

How can we tell if a new patient comes in from Snapchat or Facebook? We broadcast a different number for them to text or call, and we're able to crunch the numbers and see which platform generated the most new patients.

## Instagram

I'm on Instagram as Dr. Jeneby™ Plastic Surgeon and as Drjeneby Spa Black. My pages describe me as "Ivy League Board Certified Plastic Surgeon 15+ yrs Best of SA 8+ yrs 8,000+pts Adj. Breast Implants-Mommy Makeovers! Butt Impl/BBL."

It also refers people to my Snapchat: "Snap:drjenebytv."

Instagram, which allows you to post photos and short videos with posts and hashtags, is where we love to showcase "before" and "after" pictures of breast augs, Brazilian Butt Lifts, man boob reductions, and lipo. The photos reveal the really dramatic transformations from flat, fat, and flabby, to firm, full, and contoured.

"People really like to see Dr. Jeneby in the posts," my marketing assistant says.

So, we have several showing me undergoing the CoolSculpting procedure in Spa Black. One photo shows me shirtless, under pale blue pads and tubes, while the other half of the post image is a blonde in a red evening gown.

"At my Spa!" it says. "I get the same stuff you do! CoolSculpting my flanks, round 2! Love it!!!"

The post also says:

"Keep the Love, Lose the Handles with CoolSculpting."

Both for $1,200 now until 2/28

Photos of before and after belly

"Freeze away your fat. No Surgery. No Downtime."

#coolsculpting #drjeneby #drjenebytv #freezefat #ihatemyflanks #nodowntime #coolsculptingresults #bestofsa

Another post advertising this amazing procedure that literally freezes your fat to make it disappear, shows video of me having it done during a lunch break.

I'm lying shirtless on my stomach, and on my back are blue pads connected to tubes. The CoolSculpting King banner waves across the video. *Sometimes you gotta sacrifice!*

Blue letters stamped diagonally across the screen say, "Melt fat during your lunch!"

On the video, while the machine is working its magic, I say, "What up? We're doing my flanks one more time for the third cycle. I've had lots of good luck with CoolSculpting. We're doing a little touch up!"

Then I add, "So we've been on for a minute. It feels a little tingly, a little cold, then it gets numb. On my way to melting fat, y'all!"

Another Instagram post reflects how I'm the most expensive tailor you can hire, because I literally hem skin. We show "before" and "after" pictures with the post:

Thigh lift with Massive Weight Loss! Lipo is not enough when there is a lot of skin! A surgical thigh lift with circumferential lipo is usually required!

She also had a rhinoplasty at the same time! Past surgeries with me: Adjustable Implant with Lift/Tummy Tuck/Brachioplasty! 1.5 hours

$7,999

2-4 weeks recovery

#massiveweightloss #thighlift #rhinoplasty #drjeneby #drjenebytv #plasticsurgeon #plasticsurgery

Some other cool stuff on our Instagram pages includes:

- Me holding a four-foot Dorado that I caught on a fishing trip on the Panama Canal with my buddies.

- A pic with my sister in Dallas, where I have season tickets for my favorite team, the Dallas Cowboys.

- Me swimming with sharks in Mexico.

- Me with my staff celebrating Valentine's Day with heart-shaped pizzas for lunch.

- Super glam ads with models to promote an $8,999 Tummy Tuck Special for the holidays or a $4,599 Breast Augmentation Special.

- Video of me performing lipo on a woman's belly with a banner over the video of my fast-moving arm as the metal tube rams in and out of her flesh: "fat harvesting for BBL." That means I will inject the fat back into her butt to create a full, round behind during a Brazilian Butt Lift. Please check out the "before" and "after" pictures of this. It's really amazing how I can create something from nothing, using natural materials from the woman's own body.

- Video of a hair transplant procedure as my technician harvests hair from the back of a man's head that we will implant in his front hairline.

- The sultry, bare curve of a woman's behind—she's wearing a black thong and red high heels—to promote "BBL w/360 Lipo OR Butt Implants for $9,999."

- A picture of me in scrubs with Felix from the Billy Madison Show; he's wearing a pink surgical gown that exposes his sleeve tattoo. The hashtags say, "#makefelixhotagain and #Manover!" He was getting his man boobs removed.

All these posts show that we have so much fun while making people feel great about themselves and posting the pictures and videos for all the world to see.

## Website

The websites for my Center— https://drjenebyplasticsurgery.com/ and https://spablack.com/—are super sexy. The pages feature beautiful women wearing lacy lingerie or skimpy undergarments to show off their breasts, behinds, flat stomachs, and otherwise contoured bodies and smooth faces. All to highlight the beauty-enhancing services that we provide.

There's a blog and tons of drop-down menus where you can literally spend hours reading about all the procedures and products that we offer at the Surgi-Center and Spa.

My philosophy is that a website should be easy to use, with big numbers and all the pertinent information front and center. We have forms ready to fill out, and we offer promotions that give the visitor an incentive to fill them out.

We make it super simple to navigate and find everything you need at your fingertips.

The same goes for the Spa Black website. It lists all the services we provide, including: body contouring, dermaplaning, dermal fillers, eye treatments, facials, injectables, laser hair removal, light therapies, hair restoration, microdermabrasion, micro needling, neurotoxins, peels, skin resurfacing, and treatments for snoring and sleep apnea. We also offer acne treatments, anti-aging procedures, vaginal tightening via laser, and procedures that smooth cellulite.

Promoting the spa online generates a lot of phone calls; people call to ask questions and schedule appointments. Our social media and website may be their initial contact with us; I am obsessed with making sure that their first human contact that any caller or walk-in client has with us makes the best impression possible.

## Customer Service

Customer service and marketing are usually discussed as two different things. But I've discovered that they are equally powerful. Because bad customer service can be a marketing nightmare. How? Good, old-fashioned word of mouth advertising is the best. At one point, before I started doing Facebook Live videos in mid-2016, my marketing was 70 percent word of mouth, thanks to the large numbers of people I operated on between 2004 and 2015. I can't buy better advertising than a satisfied patient telling their friends, family members, neighbors, co-workers, and all their followers on social media that I provided an amazing procedure that changed their life for the better!

That's why I make it fun, comfortable, safe, and better beyond their expectations. I expect my staff to do the same, and we work hard to improve on our customer service every day.

Because you better believe, bad customer service is by far the worst marketing you can have for your business. If someone is treated rudely on the phone or feels disrespected by a nurse or doesn't like the way I talked to them, or worse, they will lambaste us on social media and on every doctor review website they can find. This is the double-edged sword with social media.

I make it my mission in life for the Plastic and Cosmetic Center of South Texas and Spa Black to try and provide impeccable customer service. My plastic office averages a 4.7 (out of 5.0) with 2,500 reviews!

I've been studying this like a fiend for years. In the early days of my practice, if I wasn't working, I was studying marketing and customer service.

Customer service starts when someone on my staff answers the phone. I recorded and listened to all of our incoming phone calls for three years. That was about 50-100 calls per week. If the receptionist didn't say "Hello," or if she failed to put someone on hold before asking the rest of the staff if we provide a certain service, or worse, dismissed a caller with "I don't know," I went on a rampage.

You need someone answering the phone who is sweet, knowledgeable, and who *loves* to work there.

*If you don't like being here with all the perks, GTFO!*

In my office, the receptionist (Jessica Zamora) is one of the most important people on the staff. I want her to feel good about her position. I also trust her to have her finger on the pulse of what's trending for our Center.

So, she'll give me up-to-the-minute answers when I ask: "Hey, Jessica. Are people calling? What are they asking about? What do they want? Why or why are they not signing up?"

My staff is good at this now because I coached them on how to answer the phone. The receptionist needs to feel valued in the organization, so I taught her how to represent us with the utmost friendliness and professionalism on the front lines of our business. She is the caller's first human encounter with the world of Dr. Jeneby. Callers may have seen me on videos online, and we need to continue that same upbeat vibe on the phone lines.

Now, anyone who answers our phones needs to ask the caller for their first name and last name, their phone number, email address, and how they heard about us.

I don't want my staff to only sound friendly and helpful when they realize my wife is calling. I need them to convey a cheerful, *how-can-I-help-you?* demeanor with every caller, every time. As a result, people always comment on how friendly people are in my office.

Excellent customer service is an ongoing process, from the first phone call to the discharge and throughout the follow-up. When potential new patients call us, clinical coordinators screen them, then schedule a free consultation.

If the patient passes my staff's review, then he or she is scheduled for a consultation with me, which currently costs $150. I do these on Tuesdays only. I intersperse other consults throughout the week after they have seen my coordinators. *That's tough but I love it!*

I see 1,200 people every year, on four days every month, and operate on 500 to 600 of them, which is a 40 to 50 percent closure rate. Some Tuesdays are booked with 15 to 20 new patient consults, and I spend 10 to 30 minutes with each one (they have a lot of their questions answered by the coordinator by then, and at this point, just want to meet me!). If someone is scheduled to see me, and they don't call or show up, then they are not allowed to see me again until they see a coordinator and pay a deposit.

## Success Secrets

You're probably wondering if I get sued a lot.

After all, plastic surgery might seem high risk, with a high probability of patients being unhappy with the results, or vengeful if they ended up with an infection or imperfection related to the procedure.

First, you sign several documents that describe 99.9 percent of all risks, options, benefits, and complications. You have to sign nine pages of consent forms that include your initials at the bottom. You're signing to consent for, agree to, and indemnify for almost 80 different possibilities. Then you put your John Hancock on three more documents, clearly stating that we provide no guarantees or warranties for the outcome, along with 20 other things.

The truth is, about 70 percent of patients sign and don't read it all. Only about 30 percent of patients ask questions for my staff to answer about all the waivers.

Not every outcome will be exactly how I planned it, but I feel we do an excellent job of providing informed consent. There are absolutely no guarantees in life, as well as in surgery.

But what if, on a rare occasion, something goes really wrong?

As of this writing, I have never been to court for a lawsuit. Most years, zero claims are filed against me. Other times, I may have to deal with one or two claims in a 12-month period. But I have been fortunate to not have been taken to court. Think about my schedule, with 14 surgeries per week, and 1,200 new consults a year. I'm not about to waste a single day of business sitting around in a courtroom being wrongly accused of something. I stand by my excellent work, and so do most other board-certified Plastic Surgeons around the world. At the time of this writing, I have performed more than 5,000 surgeries!

If something goes wrong, the patient really doesn't hate me. They hate that they paid money and didn't get what they wanted.

Sometimes, if something goes wrong, there's an underlying reason unrelated to the surgery. For example, I performed a breast augmentation on a young lady. She wasn't healing correctly, and I had to remove them both. Turns out, she had a genetic disorder that was interfering with her body's ability to heal.

In those rare cases, we do what's best for the patient. We resolve the problem. It also makes me feel good in these situations.

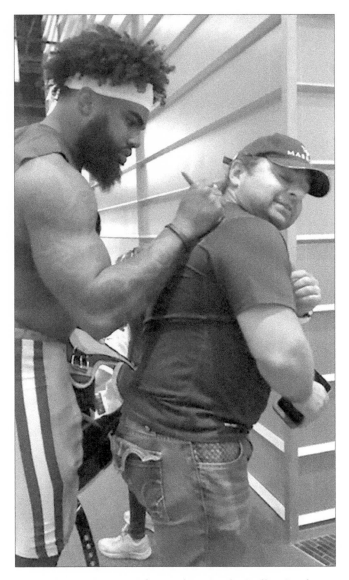

Moving to Texas meant being closer to the Dallas Cowboys;
case in point: Zeke Elliott signing my shirt!

# 7
# Philanthropy Through Plastic Surgery: The Gift of Healing and Restoring Dignity

### Becoming A Charitable Plastic Surgeon

I got involved in charitable work in Hot Springs. Early on, I started getting several calls a month with requests to donate to charities. I really wanted to give, but I wasn't sure how I could help. I didn't feel inclined to merely give money to a charity. I wanted to really change the world, but I didn't want to get caught in something where I didn't know exactly how the money was spent!

My skepticism about charities was changed with an episode of *60 Minutes* in 2003. The interviewee was a Plastic Surgeon, and the story highlighted his involvement with a women's shelter where he offered his surgical services to repair the intense and grotesque physical damage from domestic abuse these women had endured. He restored their sense of self by operating on their disfiguring scars and burns, among other things.

One hundred percent of that doc's time, money, and effort were going directly to the recipient of the plastic surgeries he did.

I was hooked on this idea.

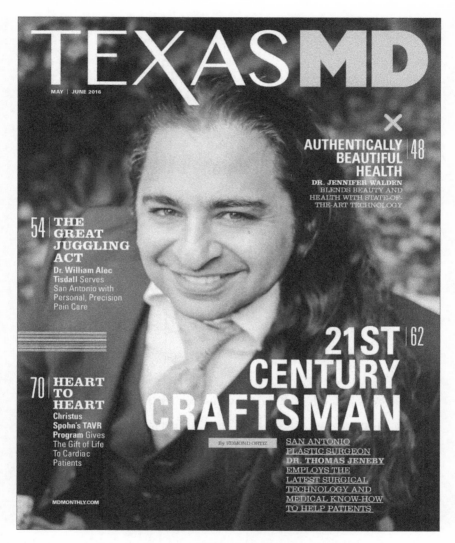

I made the cover of Texas MD magazine in 2016.

## Family Violence and Prevention in San Antonio

Deandra was a young, beautiful woman—married to an abuser. One day, he kicked her across the bedroom, and the trauma to her body caused her IUD to slice through her uterine wall. Unfortunately, she had no idea that she had suffered a grave internal wound. And for five months, she experienced internal bleeding—but didn't even know it.

Until one day, she fainted at work.

"We don't know how you're alive," doctors told her after she was rushed to the hospital.

The 25-year-old had severe sepsis—meaning that life-threatening toxins and bacteria had poisoned her bloodstream. This infection could have easily killed her.

Thankfully, several surgeries saved her life. But they left a horrific scar on her abdomen. It was 2.5 inches wide and eight inches long, circling her belly button, and making the left side of her abdomen protrude 1.5 inches higher than the right side.

"For people who have the mark of their trauma on their bodies in a way they can see every time they wake up or take a shower," Deandra said during an interview for this book, "every single instance was having to go back in time and relive exactly what happened to me."

Deandra divorced and began saving money to finance expensive plastic surgery to reduce the appearance of her scar and hopefully flatten her stomach.

She was very disturbed that the scar and her uneven belly elicited questions from children and adults every day. Some asked why she had such a large abdomen, even though she exercised a lot. Still, she felt that she could not lose the thickness around her belly.

Deandra's scarred, disfigured body was embarrassing and depressing. She tried wearing clothes that camouflaged the scar. She tried a chemical peel to diminish its appearance. And she visited Spa Black to consult with an esthetician about CoolSculpting to reduce what looked like fat on her abdomen.

"This isn't fat tissue," the esthetician said. "You have a build-up of scar tissue that is pushing your abdomen forward. How did you get this scar?"

Deandra shared what happened.

"Let me tell Dr. Jeneby your story," the esthetician said. "He's been looking for someone like you."

I had a consultation with Deandra, and she was thrilled that I would perform surgery free of charge to repair her scar. The procedure and recovery were extensive, and Deandra was immeasurably grateful that I had removed what had been a constant reminder of her trauma.

"I would've been happy with the scar the way it looked fresh out of surgery—red and puffy with the stitches in—because that was better than what I had before," Deandra said. "I could at least look at that and say, 'This was an act of kindness instead of an act of rage and cruelty.' Dr. Jeneby really did change my life."

## Survivors Have No Words

When I first ventured into helping victims of domestic violence, I called Marta Pelayo, CEO of Family Violence Prevention Services (formerly Battered Women's Shelter) in San Antonio. Two weeks after our initial meeting, I was operating on my first patient from her organization.

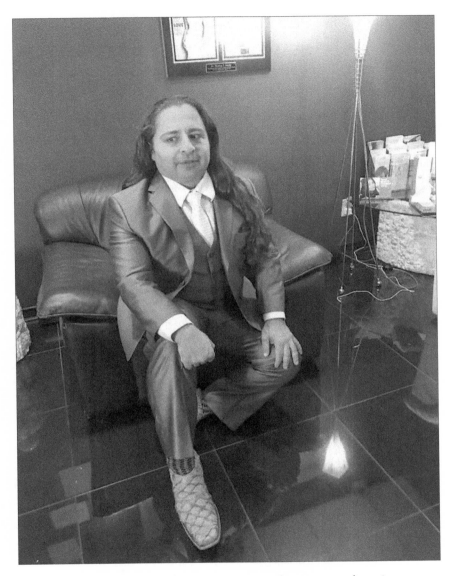

**On the set of a pilot in a great suit and even greater boots!**

After our first conversation, Marta had broken the news to two women that I would be providing plastic surgery to them free of charge. One was a beautiful, 26-year-old mother whose abuser had almost burned her alive. The scar tissue on her neck was so thick and heavy that her neck tilted—she was no longer able to hold her head up straight. The other woman had been scalped by her abuser in front of her 13-year-old son.

Marta said that when the women heard that I would help them, they were overwhelmed with gratitude. Marta recalls: "I told them, 'There is this wonderful person out there looking for candidates. Would you like to be considered?' The younger one couldn't say yes or no. She threw herself into my arms and began sobbing. Only in her wildest dreams could she imagine this."

*I am in my element.*

In addition to physical abuse, both women had suffered financial abuse by their abusers, Marta said, and as a result had no money to pay for plastic surgery, which is not typically covered by insurance.

"Thomas went in and removed the scar tissue and other repairs for [the 26-year-old mom]," Marta said. "That is critically important for her recovery. She was able to get a job working at a restaurant. She tended to her children with ease and without her kids asking, 'Mommy, why do you look that way?'"

Marta said the second candidate who had been "scalped" by her atrocious husband, "had become quite good at making all kinds of buns and twisting and teasing her hair to cover the huge gap so it wouldn't show. She never considered having something done. It was completely out of her financial range."

Rebuilding and repairing her scalp required skin grafts and several surgeries that ultimately re-connected both sides of her scalp. The woman—who is in a federal witness protection program—has written several letters expressing how her life has improved as a result of the surgery.

"It's very difficult for anyone who doesn't see these people to comprehend how these surgeries restore their dignity," Marta said. "It's not vanity. It's simple dignity."

The trauma and healing also affect their children, because in many cases, the survivors are mothers.

"Whatever the initial pain they feel," Marta said, "and their hurt, the horror, the recovery, the rehab, the benefit—it's multiplied, because it's not only impacting them, but it's impacting their children. You can imagine the woman who was scalped. Her son was 13, and he witnessed the whole thing while he lived with his mom. Now he got to see Mom happy and a different person and possibly even to lose the self-guilt that children have because Mom was no longer wearing the visible signs of abuse on her head."

Doing these surgeries has had a deep impact on me. I'm a fairly stoic doctor, trained to be tough and resilient during my surgical residency. Yet when I began to treat these patients, I was consumed by sadness and remorse.

When I first meet these women, they make no eye contact, speak in low voices, and are thankful for anything you do. It changes my frame of reference of how lucky I am to how much disgust I have for the "human being" who did this to these women.

It's deeply fulfilling to witness how the surgeries transform the women's self-esteem and give them hope and confidence to rebuild their lives. Since 2004, I have performed over 50 plastic surgeries for women who have survived domestic abuse. I now help about two to three women per month.

Once, when I was on the Billy Madison Show, a woman called in saying she needed plastic surgery due to significant injuries she suffered during domestic abuse.

"We diverted the call off the air," recalls Derek Allgood, co-host of the Billy Madison Show. "Dr. J. got with her and did a few procedures with her at no cost to help her. That call will always stand out because of Dr. J.'s reaction and how seriously he took it."

Billy Madison agrees. "You won't see in his ads that he does a lot of charity work for women who have been in domestic situations and need reconstructive surgery. He doesn't talk about it much. That's even more amazing. He does it from the kindness of his heart. It's a very nice, generous, selfless thing to do."

Helping women who have survived gruesome domestic abuse is without a doubt one of the best things that I do today.

As a result, I participate in several other charities. One is Dress for Success, a program that provides professional clothing for women who are re-entering the workforce.

## Helping Homeless People at Haven for Hope

One day after being interviewed at a San Antonio TV station, I saw Taylor Mobley, Daytime Producer for the Fox and NBC affiliates, WOAI and KABP.

She also hosts a monthly fashion segment on the San Antonio Living Morning Show. It's called Taylor'd for You, and she expanded it into an annual fashion show that raises money for local charities. Her first show benefited Dress for Success.

"I want my second Taylor'd for You fashion show to benefit Haven for Hope," Taylor told me as we chatted in the hallway before I left the station.

"I love Haven for Hope!" I said. "Count me in. I want to be involved. I love what they do."

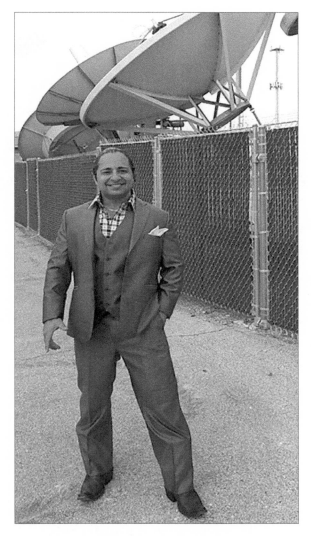

Outside NBC studios before an interview.
*Beam me up, Scotty!*

Haven for Hope is a not a typical homeless shelter. It's set up like a college campus. Men, women, and children live there and receive services that help them transform their lives to achieve indepen- dence and financial security. Hundreds of people receive: treatment for addiction; counseling; childcare; and self-empowerment pro-grams. Their goal is transformation to find long-term solutions, not just a temporary fix, for people who are homeless.

"Dr. Jeneby was my first unofficial sponsor for the second Taylor'd for Success show," said Taylor during an interview for this book. "I was super excited that he wanted to be involved. He was a platinum sponsor, the highest level of sponsorship, and he wanted to get together to do Facebook Lives to promote the event."

Taylor said my support was unique because some donors give money, then do nothing more than attend the show.

"Dr. Jeneby wanted to get the word out about the show and the cause," Taylor said. "That meant a lot to me. He brought his wife and six or eight people to the show. I gave him a seat in the front."

The event was held on June 23, 2018 at The St. Anthony, a lux-ury hotel in San Antonio, and raised $15,000 for Haven for Hope.

"It was a blessing," Taylor said. "We're already talking about his participation in the show for next year. Dr. Jeneby is really hands-on and cares about the non-profit and philanthropy work in the community. I value the friendship and relationship. I have nothing but good things to say about him."

## Supporting Fabooblicious for Sandra's Hope Foundation
*Fab-boob-licious.*

I love that name! It started as a non-profit running team that I supported for the Susan G. Komen Race for the Cure in San Antonio. I was happy to provide T-shirts and sponsor the runners.

I backed them after I was contacted by Jovahna Gonzalez, the vice president of a breast cancer awareness advocacy group in San

Antonio. I admired her commitment to helping women learn about breast cancer prevention, as well as assisting those who are enduring the challenge of treatment.

Three years ago, when Jovahna's organization launched an annual fundraiser called Hope On The Runway, I was all in. Not only does this fashion show raise money for women who are dealing with breast cancer, but it also features models of all ages who are fighting breast cancer or who are survivors of the disease.

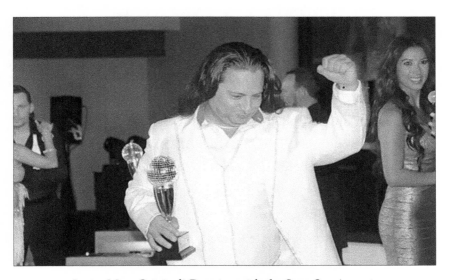

I won Most Original! Dancing with the Stars San Antonio
benefitting Family Endeavors.

"Dr. Jeneby has always sponsored the main event, the fashion show in October, which is Breast Cancer Awareness Month," says Jovahna. "Our first year was 2015, and we raised more than $10,000 that evening for our first fashion show when 150 people attended."

Jovahna—vice president of the non-profit Sandra's Hope Foundation, which is named after her friend who lost a battle with breast cancer—says she appreciates how I helped her to make this wonderful event even bigger and better.

"Dr. Jeneby really motivated me," she recalls. "He gave me ideas. And he suggested that I reach out to a local luxury boutique called Julian Gold."

As a result, the Hope On The Runway fashion show has grown tremendously. Attendance has doubled and it has become a sell-out show that moved into the upscale Tobin Center for the Performing Arts, an outdoor venue on the Riverwalk in downtown San Antonio.

"This year we raised more than $20,000," Jovahna says.

As you know, I like to help organizations where I can see how the money is being used to help people, and Jovahna is definitely doing that in a big way. So, what do they do with the money to help women with breast cancer?

"We help individuals here in San Antonio with financial assistance," she says, "whether to pay for their procedures or chemotherapies or if they're falling behind on bills, the mortgage, or the rent. We help a minimum of two individuals per month."

The organization also encourages women in the San Antonio community to learn about the importance of early breast cancer detection through screening and self-examination, and to cultivate wellness through a healthy lifestyle.

"We also provide a scholarship that comes directly from our Hope On The Runway fashion show," Jovahna says, "a scholarship for two individuals whose parents have gone through breast cancer and need assistance with their education. We provide $1,500 per student, and we've had four recipients in the past."

I also sponsor Jovahna's volleyball tournament, and some of the women from my office help out at events.

"Jetsy, who works with him in surgery," Jovahna says, "is really involved in our organization—she deejays on the side to sponsor the music. She's so sweet."

Every time she's asked me for help, I've been happy to provide it.

"There wasn't a time when he didn't say yes," Jovahna says. "He is generous with that in any small thing that we need. And he is always willing to help with the bigger sponsorships. Dr. Jeneby's generosity and compassion are the reason he does well. If you give back, you receive."

## Crowning the Chips and Salsa King

I also love charities that help children. That's why I support St. Peter-St. Joseph Children's Home for underprivileged children who have no parents.

Another favorite is SA Youth, an organization that provides a safe, after-school environment for young people who might otherwise hang out in the streets. After raising $12,000 for SA Youth, I was crowned the Chips and Salsa King for 2014. I was also given the honor of riding as King on the Fiesta Flambeau Parade float, as part of America's largest illuminated night parade that draws more than a half million people into the streets to watch the 11-day Fiesta San Antonio. That was definitely one of my top 10 moments in life.

These organizations provide the backbone for my charity life and complement my normal or otherwise busy, crazy life as a Plastic Surgeon.

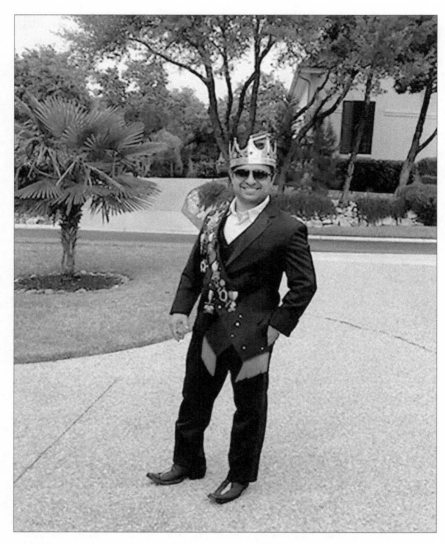

In 2014, SA Youth crowned me the Chips and Salsa King. I was also given the honor of riding as King on the Fiesta Flambeau Parade float. What an honor!

## Make Time Now

Other physicians always ask me, "How do you make time for things when being a doctor takes up 99 percent of most of our lives?"

The answer is simple: make time, and the rest of your life will follow it. I do Krav Maga and group fitness classes three times a week, fit in a massage or yoga, travel, have Dallas Cowboys season tickets, read books, and spend time with my family and friends.

Life is more than work, and balance is the key to feeling fulfilled.

My anesthesiologist told me a story in the OR one day about a urologist who used to say: "When I retire, I'm gonna do this. When I retire, I'm gonna do that." At age 50—just nearing the retirement age of this doctor—he died of a heart attack! He worked his whole life, putting off so many dreams on his I'm-gonna-do-this list, and never doing any of it!

I tell my patients this story a lot when they say, "I can't find time to eat right and exercise—just give me lipo."

I tell them all: "I'm a heck of a lot busier than you, and I find time."

Find time for charity, work, exercise, loved ones, your pets, your business. It's up to you to decide how healthy and fulfilled you're going to be. Your main priority should be your dedication to finding time to live life to the fullest. *Go get it and get it now!*

# 8
# Raving Fans

*"Success is no accident.*
*It is hard work, perseverance,*
*learning, studying, sacrifice, and most of all,*
*love of what you are doing or learning to do."*

—Pelé

Right now, thousands of women and men are walking around the world with more confidence, excitement, and success—because I helped liberate them from the shame and self-consciousness they suffered regarding their appearance.

When I perform plastic surgery on men to get rid of fat stomachs, man boobs, balding, puffy eyes that make them look old and so on, their confidence spikes. They get a peppier step. They go out. They get new jobs. They tell their old bosses to "take this job and shove it!"

Likewise, breast augmentations, Mommy Makeovers, and Brazilian Butt Lifts make women feel beautiful and their self-esteem soars.

"We call him the Hands of God," says Billy Madison, who shares his success story about his NeoGraft hair implant procedure at Spa Black in this book.

Likewise, during my weekly "Ask Dr. Jeneby Anything" spot on the Billy Madison Show, I've touched the lives of his crew and co-hosts, including his producer, Felix Diaz, and co-hosts Derek Allgood and Nathan "Nard" Norris.

"Doc is like a god in being able to craft Nard's wife's boobs," Billy says. "He might have saved Nard's marriage because of that."

A Facebook video called "Tatas for Tracy" just prior to her February 19, 2014 breast aug surgery has nearly 80,000 views.

"She's definitely topless right now in front of another guy," Nard tells someone on the phone while I markup Tracy's chest with a purple pen during the five minute, 19-second video. "He's still marking. I don't know why he has to add that many lines."

Tracy's surgery went well, and they are both happy with the results.

On the show, Nard, Derek, and Billy love to banter about how a breast aug is often a decision that couples make together, and that big boobs improve men's moods and relationships in general.

"We call them good mood boobies," Billy says. "Guys tell us, every time I see my wife, I'm in a good mood, because she got boobies."

Making men and women happy about themselves, their relationships, and their lives—what more could I ask for in terms of fulfillment from my career as a Plastic Surgeon? I'm grateful beyond words that I get to devote my life's work to helping people feel better about themselves so they can live their best lives.

I boast about their success, and they do the same for me, and I love every one of my raving fans.

## Yvonne: "Dr. Jeneby is Amazing!"

"Dr. Jeneby is the best," says Yvonne Spear of Austin, Texas. "He does amazing work. He makes people happy."

The 51-year-old wife and mother says I made her dream come true, and she's loving life as a result.

"I got my beautiful, big breasts, and I'm very happy with them," she says. "Dr. Jeneby is a character. He's amazing. He has a great sense of humor. His personality is just... if anybody doesn't like him, I don't know how that happens. He's a fun man, but he's also very professional when he needs to be. He's a respectful, pleasant man. I would recommend anybody and everybody to him. To me, he's just that amazing!"

Yvonne says she's always had small breasts and dreamed of being curvy.

"I hardly had anything," she adds. "Both my sisters were given beautiful breasts, but I was always smaller. As a kid, I had nothing. I could swim without a shirt."

Yvonne, like a lot of women, declared that when her kids reached a certain age, she would go for it.

"I always wanted a breast aug," she says now. "I was always small, but after having two babies, they got even smaller."

Even though she lives 80 miles from San Antonio, Yvonne heard about me through two high school friends at a reunion. One friend had had surgery, and one friend had just had a consultation.

"I set a date," she says. "I said, 'I'm gonna get it done this coming year,' and I did it."

That was in 2010. But Yvonne did some shopping around before coming to me.

"A friend of mine from work had a breast aug in Austin, and

she referred me to her doctor," she says. "I went to their website, read some reviews, and had a consultation. He wasn't convincing enough. He was trying to get me [to agree to] silicone implants, even though I told him I wanted saline. He said I'd get better results from silicone. I told him I was concerned with silicone leaking."

Yvonne works as a clinical manager in an obstetrics/gynecology facility and had encountered a patient with breast pain. The cause turned out to be leaking silicone from her implants.

"She got very sick," she says. "[The other doctor's] pictures looked great, but that was not what I wanted."

One of Yvonne's cousins, as well as the friend from high school, had been my patients.

"I looked him up," she says. "I looked at his website, and he had amazing results. He had great reviews. His patients spoke very well of him. So, I set up a consultation. He recommended saline. He told me about the adjustable implants. I was very interested, because I didn't know how big I wanted to go. Since they are adjustable, he can keep adding more saline into the ports until I'm happy."

Adjustable implants are my specialty. What you don't know is that after a breast aug, you are going to be swollen. You are going to be big. But when the swelling goes down, you may say, *Hey, Doc, I wanted them to stay that big.* That's called "Boobie Remorse!"

If you don't have adjustable implants, you're looking at another surgery. With adjustables, you just come back in and we add more saline until you're happy.

Yvonne came in three times after surgery. So how big did she go?

"I don't want to scare you," she warns. "Don't go by the bra number or size, but I'm wearing a 34F. That sounds like, 'Oh, my God!' but I have broad shoulders. I wanted to be proportioned to my body shape. They are perfect. They look natural and pretty. They're nicely shaped. Before surgery, I was a 32/34B, a full B. They were very saggy. They deflated after breastfeeding my two boys."

Back when Yvonne had her breast aug, I wasn't doing surgeries live on social media. But she has come back for other surgeries since, and those have been broadcast.

Thinking back on surgery, she says, "The pain was tolerable. Dr. Jeneby's team made me very comfortable. I was back to work quickly with a light schedule and no lifting. It was an easy recovery."

Yvonne is 51 years old and looks great.

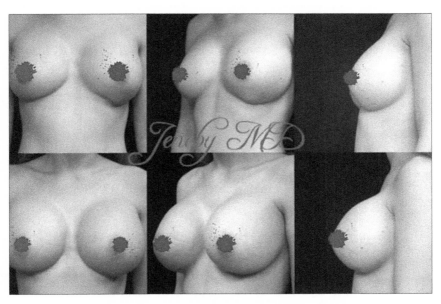

**Three adjustments in 7 months: from 32A/B to 36DDD.**

"I feel better about myself," she says. "I have more confidence. I'm very happy with my breasts. I made a good decision. I've been married to my husband for 23 years, and this has sparked up our relationship. It's a sexy thing between the two of us. It's romantic.

My husband is very supportive of my decision and we're happier now than when we were very young. We have great jobs, a family, and I have my breasts.

"My sisters got naturally huge breasts," Yvonne says. "I just did not get any. I don't know what happened. I told my mother, 'I think you gave me powdered milk, and you gave them whole milk.' Now I tease them: 'I bet if we show our boobs off, mine are standing up and yours are not.' They were supportive of me and happy for me."

Some of Yvonne's other procedures have included blepharoplasty to remove under-eye bags and a tummy tuck.

Yvonne says she inherited puffiness beneath her eyes: "My mom has them, my gramma had them, my grandpa had them. I had the fatty tissue removed. And it was live on social media. Everyone from work, friends, sisters, saw it on September 9, 2015."

Yvonne said people watching were in shock.

"People said when I went back to work, 'Oh my God, I was freaking out for you.' The pain wasn't bad, but my bruising was significant. The end results were amazing."

Yvonne got phenomenal results from her 2011 tummy tuck, too.

"The healing process [versus the breast aug] was harder," she says. "I came home with a drain, Steri-Strips, stitches, follow-ups. But it was all well worth it."

The fact that Yvonne came back for multiple surgeries is a great endorsement, and her words are meaningful. Yvonne has also come to Spa Black.

"I had laser hair removal done on my legs and underarms," she says. "I like to return for minor procedures. I don't need any more surgery."

She says I help women feel beautiful again after life takes its toll on their bodies.

"Women go through a lot," Yvonne says. "We have babies, we take care of our families, we sacrifice our bodies, and he puts them back together for us, and that's amazing. We deserve to get beautified at times. I love when he has those Mommy Makeovers. Those are amazing for the ladies who do that—they deserve it."

*Amen!*


## Shirley: "I am 55 Years Old and I Look Fabulous!"

I am alive.

I am vibrant.

I look good.

I feel good.

I look good in my clothes.

I feel good about who I am as a person.

In late 2016, Shirley Bratton's outlook on life was simple: "I'm almost 60 years old," she thought. "I'll be sitting on the porch soon, drinking lemonade, and waiting for death to knock on my door."

Fourteen months later, people don't recognize her, and that rocking-chair mindset is gone forever from her mind.

At age 54, Shirley embarked on a quest for a better life. Her January 2017 resolution was nothing unique: she wanted to get fit and lose weight, which are the top two most common New Year's resolutions.

Having been heavy her entire life, Shirley knew the burden of carrying extra weight. She also knew it was now or never.

"I had no health issues," Shirley says. "But my doctor said, 'You know what, Shirley? At the rate you're going, you're going to keep getting bigger. At your mature age, that will eventually impact your health.' Not only that, I travel a lot, and planes are getting smaller and smaller. My doctor said I needed to take a step back because the older I get, the more wear and tear on my life."

That's when Shirley decided to get serious about fitness.

"I loved myself," Shirley said, "but I could stand to lose some weight, so I joined a gym near my house. They had a challenge to lose weight and win money. I started working with a fitness trainer, and I was losing weight quickly. I started liking going to the gym."

She liked it so much, the spirit of the weight-loss challenge inspired her to declare: "I'm gonna compete in my first bodybuilding competition later this year."

She started working with a bodybuilding trainer in addition to her fitness trainer.

"I was going to compete in November," she recalls. "And my fitness trainer referred me to Dr. Jeneby because he'd worked with his nurse."

If she was going to have a competitive edge in bodybuilding, Shirley needed to look the part. She came in for a liposuction consultation.

"I thought it would be a suck here, a suck there," Shirley says, "so I could compete."

The reality of Shirley's body after weight loss and her desire to bodybuild competitively told a different story.

"When I went to Dr. Jeneby's office," Shirley says, "in my head, I'm thinking, 'I've never thought about plastic surgery.' I knew with the hanging stuff and fat I could not put on that itty-bitty bikini and walk across the stage in a bodybuilding competition."

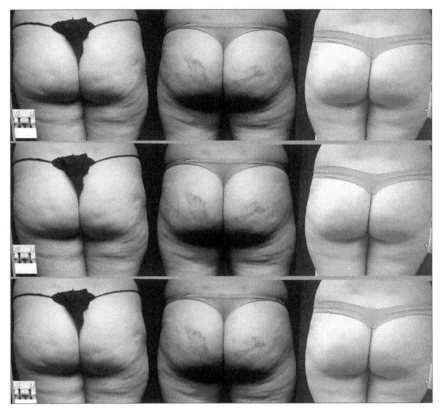

Cellfina™ for cellulite really works!

During the consultation, I confirmed that diet and exercise could not fix Shirley's hanging skin.

"You need surgical intervention," I told her.

Shirley had had an emergency abdominal surgery a few years earlier, she'd had a couple of kids, and she was working against gravity. Her loose skin was not going to snap back. Her boobs were not as perky as they'd once been.

"Lipo won't get you where you want to be," I told her. "And girls in bodybuilding have perky boobs."

My recommendation was that we wait until Shirley was at her desired weight and body fat percentage before doing anything with her breasts.

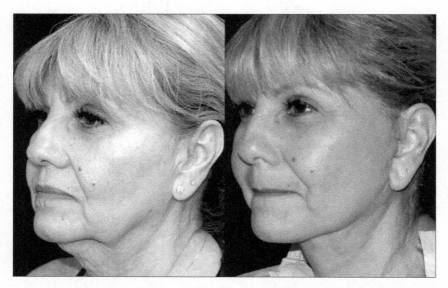

**This 57-year-old loves her face and neck after a mini facelift and a full necklift!**

"Dr. Jeneby told me, 'You probably want the implants because when you lose weight and get thinner, your boobs will shrink up even more, and when you look at competitors, you won't have that edge.'"

Shirley ran my recommendations by her trainer, and they agreed to wait until Shirley could get everything done at once. She'd be getting a Mommy Makeover.

"In December, I got a breast lift with adjustable implants, a tummy tuck, lipo on my inner thighs, under-arm lipo—side boobs, underarms, and back—and lipo in that special area above the vagina."

When I asked Shirley if she wanted her surgery broadcast live, she was skeptical, but agreed.

"Just don't show my face," she said at the time.

In retrospect, Shirley says, "I was going to keep it to myself, but I decided to do something different."

Knowing she wouldn't be recognizable, she figured it would help others who were thinking about the surgery.

Shirley's biggest fear going into surgery was her potential level of pain. The horror of her emergency hysterectomy two years earlier had her concerned about another surgery on her abdomen. That time, she woke up screaming after surgery and the morphine they were giving her did nothing to ease the excruciating pain.

Fortunately, that did not happen again.

"Immediately upon waking up from the five-hour surgery in the suite," Shirley recalls calmly, "I wasn't sure where I was. I travel a lot. When I remembered that I was supposed to have surgery with Dr. Jeneby, I thought, 'Oh, my God, something went wrong when I went under anesthesia. I feel so wonderful and relaxed and at peace with no pain.' I asked the nurse what happened. She said, 'You had surgery.'

"'Are you kidding me?' I said, flabbergasted. I had zero pain. 'I thought I hadn't had surgery because I woke up so at peace.' I've never experienced anything so beautiful in my life."

Shirley says there were moments of intense pain, but overall, she said it was a three on a zero-to-10 scale, with a few moments of eight.

As Shirley recovered, she watched her own surgery video and even read the comments, one of which was, "Is she alive?"

Shirley became enthusiastic about alleviating people's fears and concerns, not only about the surgery, but the follow-up.

"I want to let people know how I'm doing at three months, at six months, and at the one-year point, so they can see the transition. Not only is the girl alive, but she's doing well."

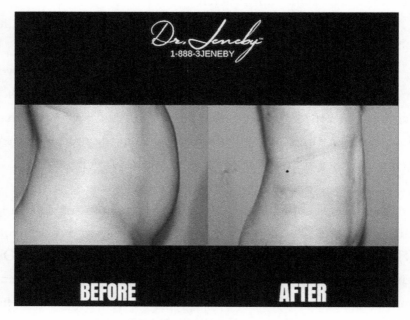

**Beautiful "before" and "after" liposuction!**

Shirley initially didn't want people knowing her business and seeing her on the operating table. Then she thought, "What if it can help or show people, and they can benefit from it?"

She then realized it's her journey to share. "I knew it would work. I felt as part of my life, I needed to share this journey. People can see my progress."

Shirley gets emotional when she thinks about the impact of this journey.

"Diet and exercise gave me weight loss," she says confidently. "Surgery enabled me to compete. But this journey has been the hardest thing I've ever done in my entire life. It has demanded everything of me: physically, mentally, emotionally, spiritually.

"The surgery was life changing," she says emphatically. "The surgery is an even higher level of life-changing than the weight loss. I always had a pooch and weight issues. When I look at myself today, I'm hot. I am 55 years old and I look fabulous.

"For the first time in my life," she says, "I wear my shirts tucked in. I don't have to wear a jacket to conceal my stomach. When I put on my jeans, tuck my shirt in, and I look at myself in the mirror, the stomach is gone. By the way, I can put on a bikini, and I've never worn a bikini in my entire life."

Shirley was confident before weight loss and surgery, but she says her self-esteem has lifted to a whole different level.

"I am a new, transformed person," she declares. "I'm revived and refreshed. People don't know I'm 55. I'm only three months out, and I still have swelling. What I look like today is frickin' crazy. It's nice to have perky boobs. I recently resumed training to build up my strength. I'm going to compete in the 'transformation' category."

Shirley says some people want Fat Shirley back.

"But Fat Shirley isn't coming back!" she declares. "This transformation has been very spiritual for me. Dr. Jeneby said it would be all right, and I put my trust in him. I am so happy and grateful. I did not know what it would do for me. My spirit and soul radiate even more, and people pick up on that. I feel holistically happy and complete in my life. I have a peace and a joy, like, *Thank you, Jesus! Thank you, God, for bringing Dr. Jeneby into my life.* Now I thank God for being able to go through this and share with other people."

### Felix: Man Boobs Be Gone!

One day when I was on the Billy Madison Show, I talked about my procedure to help men with man boobs. Producer Felix Diaz was all ears.

"I had a gynecomastia," he says. "That's female tissue where I'm supposed to have dude tissue on my chest. You want to have something in common with girls, but you don't want it to be boobs."

About six months ago, the 29-year-old came to my Center for surgery and lipo around his abdomen.

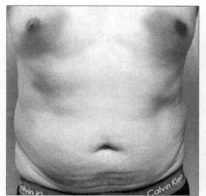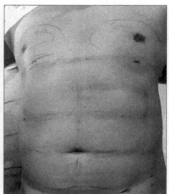

**This is Sparta! Man boob reduction and abdominal etching.** *How you like me now?!*

"It's pretty dope," Felix says now. "Not having man boobs is something super cool. I don't have to plan my clothes around man boobs. That's pretty badass. We talked about it on the air."

Felix says he didn't have much pain after surgery. But watching the video of the procedure, which I did live on Facebook and Snapchat, was hard.

"When he was doing the lipo," Felix recalls, "he's stabbing you with that super-long thing, so you're wondering, 'Holy crap! Where the hell is that going?' He wasn't doing it soft and slow."

Felix says he keeps a pretty low profile, but the surgery has really boosted his confidence and helped him get rid of the self-consciousness of feeling unattractive because of his man boobs.

"Dr. Jeneby is the best doctor I've had," he says. "He's easy to talk to. A real cool person. I'd recommend him to other guys."

He also visited my Center two years ago for me to remove a cyst on his arm.

"His staff is nice. They're all there to make sure you get to the goal you're trying to get towards."

Billy Madison says he's excited to come back to Spa Black for more NeoGraft hair transplants and tells other guys that they and their girlfriends and wives should come to me for help on whatever they need.

"Doc is witty," Billy says. "He's funny. But most important, he's just amazing at what he does. His work is phenomenal."

I stand by my work as a board-certified Plastic Surgeon who gives back to the community to help others. Every time one of my patients talks about how I've changed their life for the better, I am overwhelmed with gratitude. And when they refer new patients, I'm even happier, because that means more people will be walking around living a better life.

Life is not always a dance. Sometimes it's more like a wrestling match. If you are thinking about plastic surgery or spa stuff, go ahead and get it. Life is too short. Moms are always telling me, "I'm doing this for me now. I raised kids, got them going, and now I'm doing this for me!"

I say, "Grab the bull by the horns! You only live once!"

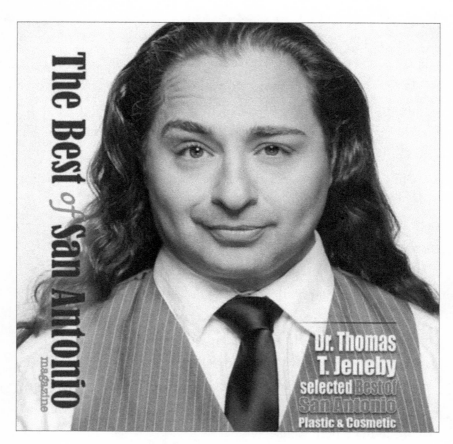

The Best *of* San Antonio magazine

Dr. Thomas T. Jeneby selected Best of San Antonio Plastic & Cosmetic

Privileged as Best of San Antonio Cover!

# Epilogue

*"A man is not a man*
*until he writes a book,*
*plants a tree,*
*and sires a son."*

—*My Grandfather*

One of the biggest reasons for writing this book has been to honor my late grandfather. PhD. Diplomat. Lawyer. All-around cool dude. My mom says I act, think, socialize, and give just like he did. An honor and a privilege to be genetically linked to him!

Truth is, I love my life. I love my staff, my patients, the solitude of the OR, the fun and philanthropic endeavors I get to participate in, and so much more.

I also want to commend Ashliegh, my beautiful and sassy wife for watching my back at all times and for raising Kallie, my step-daughter, so well.

My sister and my niece Kenzie are a blast. Mom and Dad and my cousins all thought I was crazy to do this…they were right!

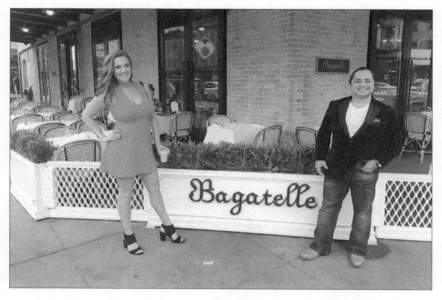

**On another adventure with Ashliegh—this time in New York City, baby!**

So, listen to my weekly live interviews on 99.5 KISS Rocks San Antonio; watch my surgeries on Snapchat, Facebook, Instagram, and Twitter; and give me a shout out!

—Dr. J.

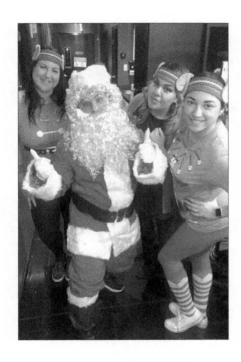

Giving back with my elves during Christmas to the underprivileged children.

Grabbing the Bull by the horns in Fort Worth Texas Stockyards.

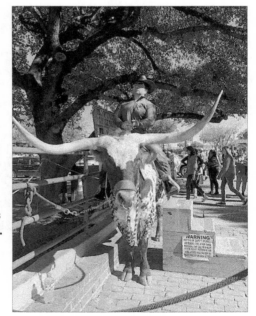

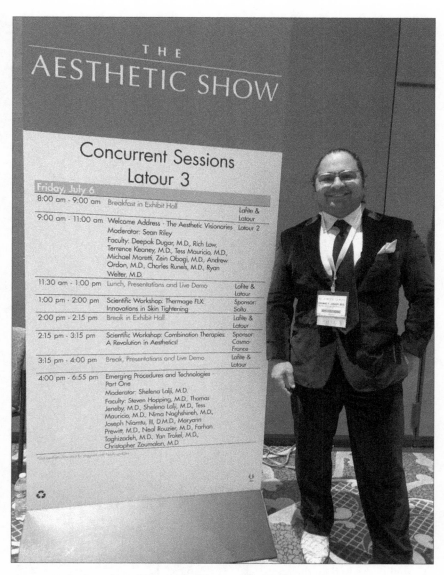

**Guest Speaking at The Aesthetic Show Las Vegas 2018.**

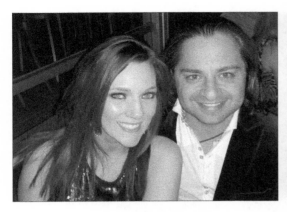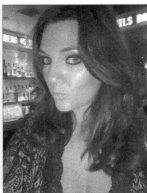

She's lovely, she's sassy… she's Mrs. Jeneby!

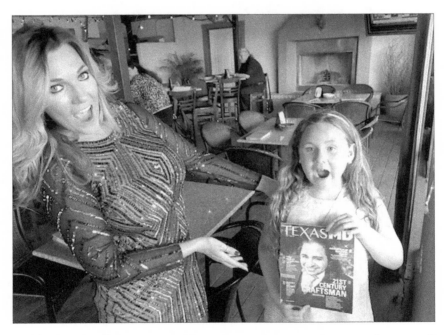

Ashliegh and Kallie expressing their excitement over my picture on the cover of Texas MD magazine. We went out on the town to celebrate.

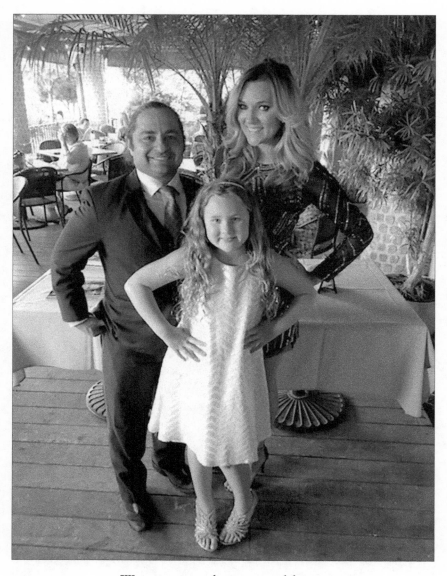

We went out on the town to celebrate.

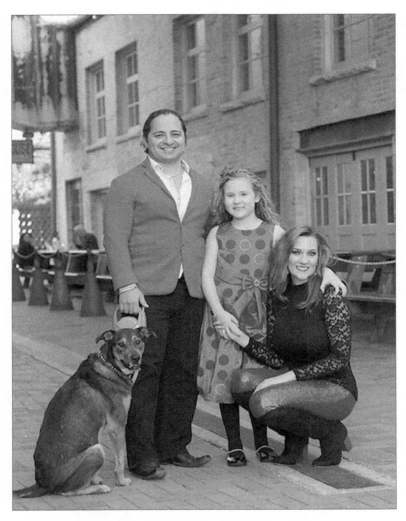

Family time in the Pearl with our dog, Venus.

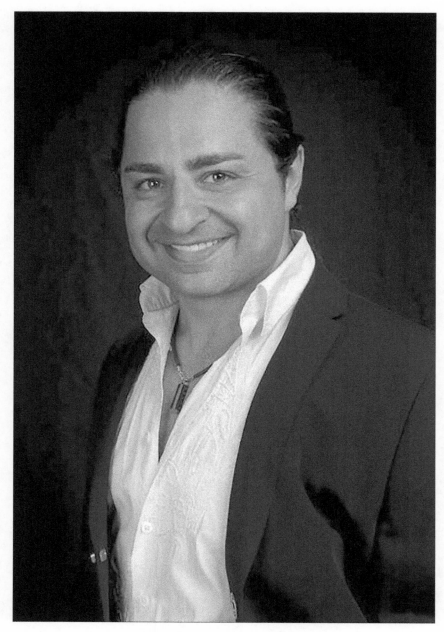

Photo Credit: Louis Scott Photography

# Biography

Dr. Thomas Jeneby is a board-certified Plastic Surgeon in San Antonio, Texas.

He obtained his medical degree from the Medical College of Virginia/Virginia Commonwealth University in Richmond, Virginia. He was featured in the top 10 percent of his class and was also in the Medical Honor Society AOA President.

Dr. Jeneby has been in practice since 2002. He has held the position as President of the San Antonio Society of Plastic Surgeons since 2016. In recognition for his performance as one of the most competent cosmetic surgeons in San Antonio, Dr. Jeneby was honored by being appointed a Diplomat of the American Board of Plastic Surgery in 2003 and recertified in 2012. He currently holds state medical board licenses in Texas, Arkansas, California, Pennsylvania, and Florida.

Dr. Jeneby has been a Best of San Antonio since 2007 and his hobbies include travel, the Dallas Cowboys, and the occasional sugar-free chocolate treat!

You can follow him on Snapchat (drjenebytv), Instagram (@drjeneby), Facebook (@DrJenebyPlasticSurgery), and Twitter (@drjeneby).

Dr. Jeneby loves to help out Family Violence Prevention Services, performing pro-bono surgery on victims of assault and family violence.

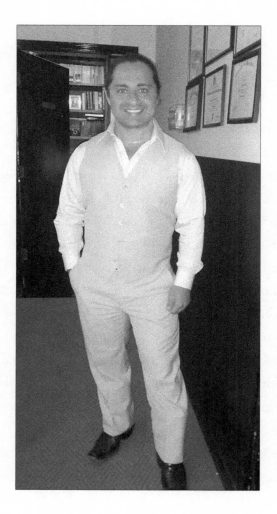

# Where to find Dr. Jeneby:

Plastic & Cosmetic Center of South Texas
Spa Black
7272 Wurzbach Road, Unit 801
San Antonio, TX 78240
Phone: 210-762-4901

## Dr. Jeneby's Social Media:

https://drjenebyplasticsurgery.com/

https://www.facebook.com/DrJenebyPlasticSurgery

https://plus.google.com/+Drjenebyplasticsurgery

https://www.instagram.com/drjeneby/

https://www.linkedin.com/company/dr—jeneby-plastic-surgery/

https://www.pinterest.com/drjeneby/

https://twitter.com/drjeneby

https://www.youtube.com/c/Drjenebyplasticsurgery

# A GIFT FOR YOU!

As a THANK YOU for purchasing
this book, I'd like to offer you
a special discount.

Bring your book to your appointment,
and you'll receive an instant discount:

- Bring in your paperback and receive:
  - ❑ $20 off spa services
  - ❑ $50 off surgery

- Bring in your hardcover and receive:
  - ❑ $50 off spa services
  - ❑ $100 off surgery

Amount Redeemed

Date Redeemed

Initials

**Disclaimer:** Must show book and gift certificate. Limit one per person. May not be combined with any other offers. Non-monetary in value. Consultation required and redemption at the discretion of Dr. Jeneby and Staff. Welcome!